Recipes My Mother Forgot

Family style cooking and a caregiver's guide to Alzheimer's Disease.

Cheryl Rhodes

Mermaid-Rhodes Publishing

Printed in Canada.

First edition: December, 1999

Canadian Cataloguing in Publication Data

Rhodes, Cheryl (Cheryl Ann)
Recipes my mother forgot

ISBN 0-9686413-0-X

1. Cookery. 2. Rhodes, Isobel, 1923 – 3. Alzheimer's disease—Patients—Biography. 4. Alzheimer's disease— Patients—Family relationships. I. Title.
TX714.R54 1999 641.5 C99-911298-8

Mermaid-Rhodes Publishing
11-5850-177 B Street
Surrey, B.C.
V3S 4J6

e-mail: mermaids@home.com

Table of Contents

Acknowledgements

I wish to thank the following people for their assistance in helping me write *Recipes My Mother Forgot*.

Mother's friends who exchanged recipes with her: Marguerite Leach, Doris Mattick, Joyce Schulz, Hollie Stothert, Kay Todd, Georgina Watson, Martha Watson, and Olive Wilson.

Kerry Murphy, Jim Rhodes, and Norma Dacre for proofreading and contributing stories. Thank you for your support.

My fellow entrepreneurs from SEEDS Group 15. Thank you for your encouragement.

This book is dedicated to my mother, Isobel Jean Rhodes.

FOREWORD

Alzheimer's Disease is the most common and best known type of irreversible dementia. Symptoms include loss of memory, difficulty with common, daily tasks, and mood and behavior changes. It affects both men and women, generally 65 years of age and older, although people in their forties, fifties, or early sixties may also be affected. At present it is estimated that over 43,000 people in the province of British Columbia, and over 300,000 people in Canada suffer from dementia. About 64% of these people have Alzheimer's Disease. In the United States about four million people have Alzheimer's Disease.

Alzheimer's Disease has a slow onset and in the early stages very few people recognize minor pauses in conversation or lapses in memory as signals of Alzheimer's. Family members may have difficulty specifying exactly when the problems began, and the symptoms may be present for many years before family and friends become concerned. In the early stages of the disease, the person is generally alert most of the time and may be aware that something is wrong, although he or she may deny there is a problem.

There is no single test that can diagnose Alzheimer's Disease. The diagnosis can take time and usually involves assessments and tests to eliminate the presence of any other medical conditions. Health care professionals look for problems with the patient's memory, use of language and expression, judgment, ability to reason, and how these affect daily functions. Diagnosis of Alzheimer's Disease comes after all other possibilities have been ruled out, and based on the judgment of a physician experienced in dealing with dementing illnesses.

Alzheimer's Disease affects a person's ability to function, affecting everything someone thinks, feels, and does. The disease affects a person's ability to remember information, remember friends and family, experience language problems, travel from one place to another in familiar areas, remember what day or time it is, plan and initiate normal, commonplace tasks, make decisions on safety issues and what to do in an emergency, difficulty eating, dressing, and bathing, and inability to control emotions. A person suffering from Alzheimer's Disease may be afraid of what is happening, become frustrated, angry, agitated, and worry about family members.

Communication becomes difficult as the person with Alzheimer's Disease may have difficulty finding the right words to use or understanding what someone else is saying to them.

A person with Alzheimer's Disease may experience difficulty with orientation. He or she may become lost in a familiar neighborhood, or unable to comprehend time-related information such as the day of the week, the season, and when it is time to eat or sleep.

Alzheimer's Disease will affect a person's judgment and thinking, often making it difficult to be aware of their surroundings and unsafe situations.

The disease affects memory, thought processes, and how someone feels, often making the patient afraid of what is happening around them. They can become frustrated, angry, or agitated, and might cry, laugh, or shout at inappropriate times.

Alzheimer's Disease affects a person's ability to perform many of the everyday tasks that most of us take for granted such as dressing, bathing, and eating.

There is no known cause for Alzheimer's Disease, although researchers have suggested several possible factors including chemical changes in the brain, a virus, environmental toxins, and genetic factors. Multiple causes have also been considered, but at the present time, no definitive cause has been determined. It is known that Alzheimer's Disease gradually destroys vital nerve cells in the brain, and the disease can only be diagnosed with a brain autopsy after death.

Since the cause of Alzheimer's Disease remains unknown, there are no recommended steps that one can take to lessen the chances of acquiring the disease. Although there are a number of medications with short term affects of delaying the onset of Alzheimer's Disease, there are no medications which will halt and reverse the disease process. Research continues, and there are several medications currently undergoing testing.

ISOBEL RHODES

My mother always had a poor memory. When I was younger she would buy candies, books, and other treats and hide them. She didn't want us to locate the treats before she was ready to give them to us but then she never remembered her hiding spot. I found Halloween fireworks stashed in the back of a cupboard in the den in the middle of the following winter. When I was eleven and travelling to England, Mother bought me a book to read on the plane and hid it somewhere, but couldn't remember where she'd put it. When I was sixteen we moved to a new house and at that time the book, *Mr. Toad's Tales*, was unearthed, with me now too old to be interested in reading it. Mother was forever misplacing her keys and glasses. She used to bribe me $1 to find her missing object. After awhile the $1 was not adequate for the time invested in the search, and I would decline her generous offer.

One of my mother's habits used to drive me crazy. She would start talking to me and cut off speaking mid-sentence, usually before the critical part. She would say: "Can you go to the kitchen and get me the…." I would hop around telling her to spit it out. She claimed I made her too nervous to remember the rest of the sentence.

As the years passed Mother's memory slowly worsened, but as she was nearing seventy years old we just wrote it off as memory loss attributed to aging. She continued to hide things and forget where they were. Increasingly she was unable to complete a sentence. She became repetitive asking us the same question or repeating the same story within a short period of time. We thought this could be due to some hearing loss because she also complained that the rest of us mumbled all the time. Her hearing was checked and there was a 25% hearing loss in each ear. My father bought her a top of the line hearing aid, which she refused to wear. We dismissed her times of confusion to being unable to hear us answer her questions.

Within a couple of years we could all see significant memory loss and confusion surrounding common tasks such as banking, cooking, and housework. She forgot names of people she had known for years, and forgot places where she had lived or traveled to. Her brother, a retired doctor from England, came out for a visit in 1995 and sensed there was a problem. A few months later Mother traveled to England to visit him and during this visit my uncle and a cousin, who is a neurologist, gave her a mini-cognitive test commonly used to diagnose the presence of Alzheimer's Disease. Their living room diagnosis was that Mother was in the early stages of the disease.

As of this time, there is no ultimate test to conclusively determine Alzheimer's Disease. It can only be diagnosed through an autopsy once the patient has passed away. Doctors take various tests for other diseases, and once everything else is ruled out the remaining prognosis is generally Alzheimer's. Mother began visiting a series of doctors. Blood tests and CT scans were taken. All the results indicated my mother was in good health, but sadly we watched her slip deeper into confusion and memory loss.

There are several forms of mini-cognitive tests consisting of thirty questions that should be answered quickly by persons with normal memory. Some of the questions are naming the day of the week, the date, the city, province, country we are in, and spelling "world" backwards. These doctors also concluded Mother was in the early stages of Alzheimer's Disease. My father retired from his job and became a full-time caregiver taking over cooking and other household chores.

In 1997 he arranged for my mother's sister in London to come and visit us, as he didn't know how much longer my mother would still be able to recognize that she had a sister. Also there was a program he wanted my mother to go on, a test for new pills for Alzheimer's patients. My parents met with the doctors and psychiatrists and it was concluded she would be a good subject for the study. Unfortunately my mother refused to have anything to do with it and became very upset when the subject was brought up. As far as she was concerned she was in perfect health and there was nothing wrong with her. Denial of a problem is a common symptom in Alzheimer's patients. We wanted to get her sister out to Canada to help influence her to go on this program. Eventually my mother did agree to participate in the study, but unfortunately all the spaces had been filled.

Persevering, we learned of a new study coming up that May, a six month test period involving several hundred Alzheimer's patients. My mother was chosen as one of the people to test a new drug called Galantamine. It was a double blind study; neither the patients nor the doctors knew who was on the placebo and who was taking the real drug. The hope is that Galantamine will stabilize a person with Alzheimer's Disease, and return some logical skills. After six months all persons in the study would be given the real drug regardless of what they had previously been receiving. We were positive my mother was taking the placebo. We did not notice any signs of improvement; in fact her mini-cognitive test scores became worse, dropping to an all time low of 15 out of 30 in November, 1997. There was also a decline in personal hygiene. She wore the same clothes everyday and stopped brushing her teeth and taking baths unless she was reminded. She forgot how to use her water pik. At this time she began to take the real Galantamine, and exhibited side effects of the real drug, namely nausea. The doctor prescribed an anti-nausea medication, and after a couple of weeks her body became used to the Galantamine, and we were able to discontinue the anti-nausea mediation.

For several months my father and I had been planning a trip to England for my mother and I would accompany her. Part of the reason was to give my father a vacation from Mother and also we felt this might be the last time Mother could visit England and still recognize her relatives. A mini-cognitive test taken the day before our January trip showed a slight increase in her score to 17 out of 30.

While in England we were able to visit my mother's brother and sister and most of my cousins. Mother was able to remember her brother and sister and their respective spouses, but the names of my cousins and their relationship to us meant nothing to her.

During the time in England she began showing some improvement in her hygiene, bathing and brushing her teeth regularly, though she still preferred to wear the same clothes each day. Another mini-cognitive test after our trip showed an improvement in her score to 20 out of 30. We felt encouraged; the experimental drug was having a positive affect.

Unfortunately this only lasted a few weeks. Mother began to slip back into lack of personal hygiene, refusal to bathe and brush her teeth, change her underwear, or any clothes, and sleep in the same clothes she wore each day. Also she would get into terrible rages of temper, swearing and screaming and being uncontrollable, again symptoms common to an Alzheimer's patient. As we neared the six month period of the real Galantamine, and the one year anniversary of entering the program, my father decided to remove Mother from the study. He was hoping by getting her off the drug the mood swings would lessen. I knew mood swings were consistent with Alzheimer's Disease and could continue without the experimental drug. Also, even if the drug did not help Mother, perhaps what the doctors learned in studying her would help someone else suffering from this terrible disease in the future.

The day of the hospital visit, a complete physical and mini-cognitive test, and after consultation with the doctors, Father decided to continue the treatment. Her mini-cognitive test had fallen to 17 out of 30 again, but the doctors were convinced there was some benefit for continuation of the drug. My mother was still able to play the piano and play tennis, which may not have been possible without the drug. The doctors also prescribed a mild sedative for daily usage, and that controlled her rages.

Father was able to receive some assistance available to families of Alzheimer's patients. This included a support group, a respite volunteer, and a housecleaner/babysitter who would come for a few hours every two weeks. Mother also attended an adult daycare for Alzheimer's patients twice a week. Every second weekend Mother went to a respite centre in Vancouver, part of a hospital but run more like a hotel for Alzheimer's patients. These all gave my father a much needed rest from the 24 hour daily shifts he spent with my mother.

It was at the weekend respite centre in late August of 1998 that we had a major setback in Mother's condition. She suffered a stroke, lost the use of her right arm and leg, and is now confined to a wheelchair.

Mother was already on a waiting list for a permanent intermediate care home and after the stroke we changed our first choice to an extended care home that handles patients in wheelchairs. After two months in the hospital, she was transferred to her current residence. After consultation with the family doctor, Father made the decision to remove Mother from the Galantamine study.

Although Mother has regained some use of her right arm and hand, she is unable to walk, and rarely talks. When she does speak, mostly it is unintelligible. She doesn't usually recognize us, and seems oblivious whether we are there or not. She is entering the final stages of Alzheimer's Disease. She is in a very good residence, with plenty of activities for the seniors, and doesn't appear to be unhappy. She still enjoys music, and every week there are musical entertainers at the home. We bring videos for her to watch, and the other residents also enjoy these movies.

My mother was an excellent cook, and enjoyed preparing gourmet meals, and planning dinner parties. Her first collection of recipes was kept in a semi-hardcover 9" x 6" book with *RECIPES* written on the cover page. On the inside cover is a handwritten note: "To Darling Isabelle. New Years Day, 1950". The person who gave her this book didn't sign her name, but I'm guessing it was a gift from her sister. She wrote her recipes by hand, then typed them out years later as she constantly added to her collection with recipes from friends. Most of the pages from the handwritten recipe book are missing. Mother most likely threw away the original handwritten recipes after typing them out.

In-between the few remaining pages of her original cookbook are newspaper clippings with recipes (none of which are included in this book), household hints, a Christmas light tour, plans for a Christmas party, exercises, a list of books she wanted to read, and a notation on the movie *Seven Years In Tibet*. I took Mother to see this movie around the same time she began to take the real Galantamine. She must have written out a reference to remind herself, wrote in red ink "Don't throw out", and stuck it into her old recipe book. That was probably the last time she went into this old book.

Unfortunately, some recipes will be lost forever. There were a couple of recipes in her original handwritten recipe book that were not part of her typed cookbook. Overlooked when she was originally transcribing the recipes onto a word processor. I was able to resurrect Orange Rice and Italian Green Peppers and include them in this book. A couple of other recipes I didn't recognize, but they were either incomplete or illegible. My mother had terrible handwriting, most of her words ending in a scribble.

Recipes My Mother Forgot is a compilation of the meals she cooked for us for many years. In the mid-nineties she lost her ability to cook, and eventually forgot all the recipes that she had collected. This book provides great family style meal ideas and offers a family member's insights on the progression of Alzheimer's Disease.

Mother was born in Glasgow, Scotland on October 7, 1923. She has an older sister, Suzanne, and a younger brother, John who live in England. Mother attended Dumfries College and became a teacher. She immigrated to Canada in 1955 where she first taught school in Sherbrooke, Quebec. She moved to British Columbia in 1957 and taught school at Point Grey High School in Vancouver and Langley Senior Secondary High School until 1960. She married Jim Rhodes on December 20, 1958 and they lived in Cloverdale until 1990 when they moved to White Rock. She enjoyed painting, skiing, playing the piano, playing tennis and badminton, and was a member of a weekly bridge club.

These are my mother's recipes, and this is her story, beginning in her hometown of Glasgow, Scotland to her current residence in White Rock, British Columbia.

SOUPS

Ten Warning Signs That Could Indicate the Presence of Alzheimer's Disease

1. Memory loss of recent information
2. Difficulty performing familiar tasks
3. Loss of language expression and comprehension of speech and writing
4. Mild confusion of time, place, and identity
5. Poor or decreased judgement
6. Difficulty making decisions and plans
7. Misplacing things
8. Personality changes
9. Mild errors in judgement and calculation
10. Seeking and preferring familiar surroundings

The Reisberg Scale categorizes Alzheimer's Disease into seven stages. Stage 1 is the regular skills and abilities of a normal adult. In other words, all the population is at Stage 1 of Alzheimer's Disease. The mystery is who will develop the other stages.

Most patients crossover between the stages, often showing characteristics of two to three stages of Alzheimer's at the same time, and as we learned more about the disease we noticed this with Mother.

During 1995 some symptoms of Alzheimer's Disease were noticeable with Mother. My Aunt Anne and Uncle John, a retired physician from England, came for a visit in May, 1995. During this time Uncle John advised Father that there were symptoms of dementia present and that Mother should undergo a complete neurological examination. In November, 1995 Mother traveled to England to visit her relatives. Uncle John and my cousin Gavin, a neurologist, did a living room diagnosis during her visit, and confirmed the likelihood of early Alzheimer's Disease.

CREAM OF ZUCCHINI AND ALMOND SOUP

Here's a different way to way to prepare zucchini.

1 large onion, finely chopped
3 tbsps. unsalted butter
3 small zucchini, sliced thin (4 cups)
½ cup slivered almonds
4 cups chicken broth
½ cup ground almonds
¾ cup whipping cream
1 tbsp. brown sugar
1 tbsps. Amaretto liqueur
¼ tsp. ground cinnamon
¼ tsp. fresh grated nutmeg

In large saucepan, cook onion and butter over moderate heat for five minutes or until softened. Add zucchini and slivered almonds, stirring for five minutes or until zucchini is barely tender. Add chicken broth and simmer for 25 minutes or until mixture is reduced by one third. Add ground almonds and simmer for 10 minutes. Stir in whipping cream, brown sugar, Amaretto, cinnamon and nutmeg. Continue to cook over low heat, stirring, until soup is heated through. Serves six to eight.

One day in the summer of 1994 I came home from work to find the contents of the deep freezer defrosting on my carpet. Fish, meats, pies, berries, jams, and other formerly frozen foods were now puddling in a sticky goo on the carpet. Mother had gone downstairs to defrost the freezer, took everything out, then walked away and forgotten about it. When I came home a few hours later I was stuck cleaning up the mess and throwing everything away.

FRENCH ONION SOUP

Transform these few ingredients into a great starter.

4 large onions, finely sliced
2 tbsps butter
2 tbsps. flour
2 cans bouillon soup
2 cans water
½ tsp. pepper
½ tsp. mace
toasted bread rounds, to taste
grated cheese, to taste

Fry onions in butter until browned, but don't burn. Stir in flour. Mix well until flour is browned. Add bouillon and water. Simmer thirty minutes. Add pepper and mace. Top with toasted bread rounds and sprinkle with grated cheese.

In December 1994, my parents rented a home near Phoenix, Arizona. During their stay Mother purchased a new, very expensive tennis racket. Several months later the tennis racket went missing, and we have no idea what happened to it. My father posted a "LOST" poster at the tennis club in case Mother had left the racket there and someone had taken it home for safekeeping. A likely scenario is that Mother put the racket on the roof of her car and drove off. Mother was convinced that someone had stolen the tennis racket. We're not so sure that it was stolen. It's just as likely that Mother misplaced the racket. Father went to a sporting goods store, purchased an identical racket, and gave it to Mother. Eventually she forgot the whole incident. Mother was in the early stages of Alzheimer's at this time and this incident is characteristic of Stage 3 of the disease.

ICY CUCUMBER SOUP

Family and guests will welcome a pretty, cool dish to begin a summer meal.

3 large cucumbers, sliced
3 tbsps. butter
3 tbsps. flour
squirt of onion juice
½ cup whipping cream
2 tbsps. chopped fresh chives
salt, pepper to taste

Sauté the cucumbers in butter over low heat for approximately 10 minutes. Season flour with salt and pepper to taste, then sift over cucumbers. Gradually stir in chicken broth and onion juice. Cover and simmer for 15 minutes, then put in blender and chill. Just before serving, stir in unwhipped cream and sprinkle chives on top. Serves four. (One hour preparation.)

PARTY SOUP

A different combination of subtle flavors.

2 cans cream of celery soup
2 cans cream of asparagus soup
2 cans shrimp
1 can chicken broth
500 ml. coffee cream
½ bottle dry white wine

Mix all ingredients except wine, and heat till boiling. Remove from heat, add wine and serve. Serves twelve.

PUREE OF CARROT SOUP INDIENNE

Spicy and satisfying, a soup that is great for a cold day.

1½ pounds carrots, sliced (about 5 large carrots)
1 stalk celery, sliced
¼ medium onion, chopped
5 cups water
1 cup milk
1½ cups light cream
½ to 1 tsp. salt
1½ tsps. curry powder
¾ tsp. ground coriander
½ tsp. ground cumin
Pinch cayenne pepper
Pinch garlic powder

In saucepan combine carrots, celery, onion, and water. Bring to a boil. Reduce heat, cover and simmer for 45 minutes or until carrots are tender. Remove from heat and allow to cool for 15 minutes. Puree in blender or food processor, in batches, until very smooth and thick. In large saucepan, combine puree and remaining ingredients. Place over low heat and heat through. Serves six.

On June 26, 1996 Mother saw a neurologist for an examination for short-term memory loss. He arranged for Mother to take a blood test, E.E.G., and CT Scan. On August 21, 1996 my parents were advised the results were all normal. Unfortunately, this was the bad news because it ruled out any other illnesses that could cause the memory loss. Mother retained this information, and over the next year told everyone that the "head guy" told her nothing is wrong and that she is in good shape. On October 1, 1996 a hearing test showed a hearing loss of 25%, which may have accounted for some of her confusion. Unfortunately, the Alzheimer's Disease was rapidly progressive over the next year.

SALADS

DIAGNOSIS OF ALZHEIMER'S DISEASE

Doctors are able to diagnose Alzheimer's Disease reasonably well after a clinical assessment. This consists of a consultation with the family doctor or a neurologist. The doctor asks the patient and family members and close friends to describe what has been happening, and how the patient is currently functioning, compared to how the patient functioned in the past.

The doctor will be looking for answers to questions such as:

- What problems have been noticed with the patient?
- When were the problems noticed?
- Are the problems always present, or do they come and go?
- Is there a history of problems with the patients memory?
- Have there been personality changes or behavior problems?
- Does the patient have trouble knowing the date?
- Have there been signs of depression, paranoia, hallucinations, or delusions?

If the doctor suspects a diagnosis of probable Alzheimer's Disease, the doctor will also have the patient undergo a series of laboratory tests to see if the observed problems may be caused by another medical condition.

Some of the tests include:

- A blood count to check for vitamin deficiencies
- A blood chemistry panel to check for kidney and thyroid problems.
- CT scan or MRI to check for brain tumors, strokes, or other dementing brain conditions.

Once the doctor has determined there are no other diseases that account for the loss of memory and behavioral and personality changes, an interview is set up with the patient to assess cognitive competence. The doctor will test recent and long term memory and might ask questions such as:

- What is the date?
- Who is the Queen of England?
- When was World War II?
- What is your birthday?
- When were you married?
- What are the names and ages of your children?

The doctor may ask questions to assess the patient's judgement. For example, what would you do if you're inside a burning house? A normal person would say leave the house or call the fire department. A person with Alzheimer's might say: "I don't know" or "Stay in the house".

Following this assessment the doctor then recommends the patient to a specialist in dementing illnesses and a mini-cognitive test to assess mental function is administered. A common test consists of 30 questions. See page 118 for an example of this test.

If a full clinical assessment points to Alzheimer's Disease, it's always wise to get a second opinion and have the tests repeated by another physician, typically a neurologist who specializes in dementing illnesses.

Doctors, scientists, and researchers are constantly developing new tests to assist in the diagnosis of Alzheimer's Disease. Although there are a number of exciting developments in this area, there are currently no tests that are definitively diagnostic, nor have they been in use long enough to establish a track record.

ADmark Assays, from Athena Neurosciences, Inc., has developed a new test based on the biochemical markers tau protein and beta-amyloid42. These are proteins that appear in the cerebrospinal fluid surrounding the brain and spinal cord. Compared with persons whose brains function normally, Alzheimer's Disease patients have high levels of tau protein, more than 420 picograms/ml, and very low levels of beta-amyloid42, less than 1,240 picogram/ml. These levels are determined by performing a spinal tap. The company claims that in people over 60 years old, their test can diagnose or rule out Alzheimer's Disease with up to 95% accuracy.

Another possible Alzheimer's Disease test is based on dilation of the pupil of the eye. In routine opthamologic exams using the chemical tropicamide on 32 people who did not have Alzheimer's Disease, it had no effect on the pupils of 30 people. But it dilated the pupils of 18 out of 19 people who have Alzheimer's Disease. However, when the Mayo clinic attempted to duplicate this study, using 20 people with Alzheimer's Disease, and 20 people with normal cognitive levels, they found no differences in pupil dilation between the two groups. So although the pupil dilation test with the chemical tropicamide might have some merit, the Mayo study casts significant doubt on it.

In February, 1996, University of Kentucky researchers made headlines with a study suggesting that analysis of people's writing ability during their twenties could predict their development of Alzheimer's Disease 60 years later. Their study involved 93 nuns who joined the Sisters of Notre Dame in the 1920's. Upon entry, each Sister wrote an autobiography, which the Order archived. Sixty years later almost one-third of the nuns had been diagnosed with Alzheimer's Disease, which the researchers concluded similar to the percentage of the general population. Fourteen nuns had died, and brain autopsies were performed revealing five of the deceased nuns had Alzheimer's abnormalities. The researchers evaluated the archived autobiographies without knowing who had written the essays. They based their evaluation on language ability, idea expression and grammatical complexity. The scientists judged nine essays to be packed with ideas and grammatically complex, and considered five to be poorly written and grammatically simple. They linked each of the nuns to her autobiography. Of the nine who had well written essays, none had developed Alzheimer's Disease, but the five nuns whose essays were concluded simple had all succumbed to the disease. The researchers suggested that young-adult handwriting samples might predict later development of Alzheimer's Disease with 90 percent accuracy. However, other researchers have raised doubts to this theory, particularly surrounding the evaluative criteria, citing grammatical simplicity was related to poor cognition among surviving nuns, not to development of Alzheimer's Disease. Another objection is the sample size, only five out of ninety-three nuns with autopsy-confirmed Alzheimer's Disease. The number of cases is not enough to reach conclusions. Although it is possible that language ability during young adulthood may have some value in predicting and diagnosing Alzheimer's Disease later in life, it is far from proven.

In a small number of families, Alzheimer's Disease strikes just about everyone at an early age, during their forties and fifties, pointing to a genetic cause. Researchers have identified genetic abnormalities on three chromosomes that appear to cause Alzheimer's Disease.

- Chromosome 1: Three large families have been identified with a specific mutation of the STM2 gene on this chromosome. Family members generally developed Alzheimer's before age 60.
- Chromosome 14: 100 families have been identified with a mutation of the S182 gene, causing them to develop Alzheimer's Disease early in life, between 30 and 55 years old.
- Chromosome 21: People with an abnormal APP gene (amyloid precursor protein) on this chromosome begin to develop Alzheimer's Disease between age 40 and 65, and about 20 families have been identified with this mutation. Also, people with Down Syndrome have an extra copy of chromosome 21, and an extra APP gene. If they live long enough, virtually all people with Down Syndrome will develop Alzheimer's Disease.

A new urine test that might diagnose Alzheimer's Disease has been developed by Nymox Pharmaceutical Corp. of Montreal, Quebec. The test measures urine concentrations of the AD7C neural thread protein, which is high in patients with Alzheimer's. Testing of patients found an average level of neural thread protein at 2.3 ng/ml, compared with levels around 0.83 for healthy control subjects. The test is 80% accurate in picking up Alzheimer's Disease, and has been correctly negative about 90% of the time. This is a new test, but is available commercially and physicians are using it to assist in a diagnosis of Alzheimer's Disease. Nymox is in the process of developing another test, which is more advanced and quicker than the AD7C test.

Some illnesses leading to dementia may be treatable, and it is advisable that a diagnosis be determined as early as possible. People with symptoms of dementia should consult a doctor for a complete medical evaluation including:

- Medical history (what are the problems, how long they've been present, and when did they start).
- Personal history (what person did for a living, hobbies, any other family member who had similar problems).
- Information provided by family or close friend.
- General and neurological examinations.
- Laboratory tests (blood counts, urinalysis, thyroid tests).
- Assessment of mental functioning (memory, language, judgement, reasoning abilities).

BEANS AND GREENS

This is a main dish winter salad. Broil grated cheese over whole wheat bread and serve as an accompaniment.

1 cup dried small white beans
2 tsps. olive oil
1 tsp. Dijon mustard
2 cups loose packed fresh spinach
1 large onion, chopped
3 tbsps. lemon juice
1 garlic clove, crushed
pepper to taste

Place beans in large bowl. Add four cups water and let soak overnight at room temperature. Drain. Place beans and onion in saucepan with four cups water. Simmer until beans are tender but not mushy, about one and a half to two hours. Drain beans and place in large bowl. Whisk together oil, lemon juice, mustard and garlic. Add to hot beans. Cover bowl and refrigerate until chilled. Tear spinach into bite-size pieces and add to beans. Toss. Season with pepper. Serves four.

During 1996 and 1997 Mother would go shopping and purchase the same item several days in a row, buying more than required. She constantly made out lists and either lost or forgot them.

BROCCOLI PASTA SALAD

Serve with fillet of snapper, or sole, or serve with soup. Good winter eating.

500 gr. macaroni or medium shells
¼ cup fresh lemon juice
¼ tsp. ground pepper
1 tsp. salt, or to taste
1 whole pepperoni skinned and cut into ¼ inch pieces
1 medium green bell pepper, cut into ½ inch pieces
⅓ cup sliced ripe black olives
⅔ cup vegetable oil
2 tbsps. red wine vinegar
1 tsp. dried oregano
3 cups broccoli flowerets
6 oz. mozzarella cheese cut into ½ inch pieces
½ cup chopped red onion
½ cup chopped carrot

Cook pasta in large amount of boiling salted water until tender. Drain and rinse with cold water. Drain well. Whisk oil, lemon juice, vinegar, salt, oregano and pepper together. Set aside. In large bowl combine pasta, broccoli, pepperoni, mozzarella, bell pepper, onion, carrot and olives. Add dressing and toss to blend. Add more salt, pepper or lemon juice to taste, if needed. Serves eight to ten.

HARLEQUIN SALAD

A cool, colorful treat.

1 can crushed pineapple
1 small bottle (5 oz.) maraschino cherries
¾ cup shredded almonds
1 small bottle (3 oz.) stuffed olives
2 packages orange Jell-O powder

Drain juice from pineapple, olives, and cherries. Combine juices and add enough water to make 4 cups liquid. Heat to boiling, add Jell-O powders and dissolve. Chill until almost set. Add sliced cherries, olives, pineapple, and almonds. Turn into ice water rinsed mould and chill until set. Serves eight to ten.

> A former politician and businessman, Father knew the importance of keeping files and in 1996 began documenting Mother's behavior and the various tests she underwent.

HOLIDAY CRANBERRY MOULD

A Thanksgiving or Christmas specialty that brings color to your table.

1 envelope unflavored gelatin
½ cup cold water
1 cup salad dressing
1 package (125 gr.) cream cheese, room temperature
2 tsp. grated orange rind
2 cups fresh cranberries
2 cups boiling water
1 peeled orange
1 unpeeled orange
1 apple cored and peeled
¼ cup sugar
1 package (85 gr.) lemon flavored Jell-O
1 package (85 gr.) cherry Jell-O

Soften gelatin in cold water and dissolve over low heat. Gradually add salad dressing to softened cream cheese, mixing until well blended. Stir in gelatin and grated orange rind. Pour into 2 quart (2 litre) mould. Chill until firm. Grind together cranberries, oranges and apple in food processor. Stir in sugar. Dissolve cherry and lemon Jell-Os in boiling water. Chill until slightly thickened. Fold in cranberry mixture. Spoon over molded salad dressing cheese layer. Chill until firm. Unmold and surround with watercress, or other garnish of your preference. Serves eight to ten.

In May, 1997 Father began communications with the local case manager of the Continuing Care Division of the Ministry of Health and Ministry Responsible for Seniors in order that a file could be commenced on Mother.

INDONESIAN RICE SALAD

Extra spice adds zest to this Eastern delicacy.

¾ cup brown rice, cooked and cooled
3 green onions, diagonally sliced
2 cups fresh bean sprouts
1 cup toasted cashew nuts
½ cup light currants
1 small red bell pepper, cored, seeded, and thinly sliced
2 tbsps. toasted sesame seeds

Tamari nut dressing

4 tbsps. vegetable oil
2 tbsp. tamari sauce (or substitute teriyaki sauce)
2 tbsps. smooth peanut butter
1 tbsp. lemon juice
1 tbsp. wine vinegar
1 clove garlic, crushed
2 tbsps. honey
1 tsp. (or more, to taste) curry powder
¼ tsp. ground ginger
pinch black pepper

In a large bowl combine rice, onions, bean sprouts, cashews, currants, red bell pepper and sesame seeds. Make the dressing in a separate bowl. Beat together the oil, tamari sauce, peanut butter, lemon juice, vinegar, garlic, honey, curry powder, ginger and pepper. Pour the dressing cover the salad and toss to combine well. Cover and marinate in the refrigerator for 30 minutes to one hour before serving.

Serves twelve.

LENTIL AND BROWN RICE SALAD

A wonderful way to use leftover rice, this salad makes a great lunch.

2 cups water
½ cup brown lentils
½ tsp. salt
1 cup brown rice
1 medium onion, chopped
2 tbsps. lemon juice
2 tbsps. vinegar
½ cup vegetable oil
1 clove garlic, crushed
½ tsp. coriander
1 cup diced cucumber
3 tbsps. chopped parsley
2 medium tomatoes, peeled seeded, and chopped
2 green onions, chopped

Combine water, lentils and ¼ tsp. of salt in saucepan. Bring to boil. Cover and simmer until lentils are tender, about 30 min. Drain well.

While lentils are cooking, cook rice according to directions.

Combine rice, lentils, and onion in serving bowl. Blend lemon juice, vinegar, oil, garlic, coriander and remaining ¼ tsp. salt. Add to rice mixture, mixing well. Chill. Just before serving add remaining ingredients and mix well. Serves six.

ORANGE AND APPLE SALAD

Good with roast pork or pork chops.

2 oranges, peeled and cut into bite-sized pieces
½ cup celery
1 to 2 tsps. brown sugar
1 red apple, cut into bite-sized pieces
¼ cup raisins
1 tbsp. fresh lemon juice.

In bowl combine all ingredients. Chill. Serves four.

THREE BEAN SALAD

For best results, prepare a day in advance and chill overnight.

1 can (398 ml) cut green beans, drained
1 can (398 ml) cut wax beans, drained
1 can (398 ml) kidney beans, drained
1 green pepper, chopped
1 onion, chopped or sliced
¾ cup sugar
½ tsp. black pepper
½ cup salad oil
1 tsp. salt
½ cup vinegar
½ tsp. Worcestershire sauce

Combine beans, pepper, and onion. Mix dressing ingredients together. Pour over beans and toss. Chill overnight. Drain. Serves six to eight.

One can garbanzo beans can be added if desired.

TOMATO ASPIC SALAD

Brighten your meal with this colorful salad.

2 cups tomato juice
1 bay leaf
1 small onion, sliced
dash of pepper
½ tsp. salt
3 oz. package gelatin
2 tbsps. vinegar
1-2 cups diced cooked vegetables (your choice)

Combine tomato juice, bay leaf, onion, pepper, salt. Heat to boiling. Strain. Dissolve gelatin in hot liquid. Add vinegar and chill until slightly thickened. Fold in vegetables. Chill until firm. Serves six.

WILD RICE SALAD

Donated from Mother's friend, Hollie Stothert.

1 cup rice (or combine ½ cup wild and ¼ cup brown)
2 tbsps. lemon juice (or more to taste)
can of cashew nuts (or amount that you like)
1 cup celery, finely cut
¼ - ½ cup mayonnaise, to taste
1 small jar pimentos, mashed fine
1 can (227 ml) water chestnuts
1 large bunch green grapes
2 green onions, finely chopped

Cook rice, and when sufficiently cool, add the rest of the ingredients. Feeds a lot of people.

VEGETABLES

STAGE 2: VERY MILD COGNITIVE DECLINE

Stage 2 of Alzheimer's Disease is the very beginning of the disease, and can be difficult to notice in some adults as they still function at a very normal level for an adult of their age group. During a clinical interview there may be no objective evidence of memory deficit, and the patient might not show any deficit at their place of employment or in social situations. This is the beginning of very mild cognitive decline and forgetfulness. The patient may complain of some memory deficit such as forgetting where they have placed a familiar object or forgetting names they formerly knew well.

Other symptoms that may be present are:

- Verbal outbursts
- Some tearfulness
- Anxiety
- Agitation
- Beginnings of suspicion and paranoia

ALMOND RICE PILAF

Leftovers can be used for vegetable pie crust.

1 cup brown rice
½ cup chopped onion
2 tbsps. toasted sliced almonds
2 cups chicken stock (or vegetarian stock)
2 tbsps. chopped fresh parsley
2 tbsps. grated Parmesan cheese
parsley sprig

Wash rice well under cold water. Bring stock to boil in medium saucepan and add rice, onion, and parsley. Reduce heat and cook, covered 45 minutes, until done. Mix in almonds and cheese. Garnish with parsley sprig.

BAKED BEANS

This recipe came from Mother's friend and bridge club member, Olive Wilson.

2 cups small white beans
2 tbsps. molasses
1 tbsp. brown sugar
1 tsp. dry mustard
4 tbsps. ketchup

The night before, put beans in pot and cover with water. The following morning bring to a boil and simmer for 5 minutes. Leave for an hour. Mix all ingredients in casserole or bean pot and place in 250 ° F oven and cook for 4-6 hours. Serves four.

Non-vegetarian version: Cut ham into pieces and add to bean pot.

BROCCOLI SUPREME

A pretty side dish to accompany your main entrée.

24 oz. frozen or fresh broccoli
2 eggs, beaten
1 cup cottage cheese
1 - 2 tbsps. grated cheese
1 tsp. minced onion
½ tsp. pepper
1 tsp. Worcestershire sauce
2 tbsps. melted margarine or butter
¼ cup dried breadcrumbs
2 tbsps. margarine

Cook broccoli until tender. Drain well. Arrange in a greased casserole.

Combine eggs, cottage cheese, grated cheese, onion, pepper, Worcestershire sauce, and melted butter or margarine. Pour over broccoli. Top with breadcrumbs and margarine and bake in the oven at 350° F for 30 minutes till golden brown.

CANDIED SWEET POTATOES

Sprinkle with chopped pecans to add crunch.

8 medium sized sweet potatoes or 2 cans (540 ml) of Yams
1¼ cup brown sugar, firmly packed
⅓ cup orange or pineapple juice
¼ cup butter or margarine

Boil potatoes until tender, then peel and halve (or use canned yams, drained). Arrange in buttered bake dish. Mix sugar and fruit juice, add butter, and bring to boil. Pour over potatoes. Bake uncovered in 375° F. oven 20 to 25 minutes, basting occasionally. Serves eight.

COPPER PENNIES

An interesting color and taste sensation.

2 pounds carrots
½ cup chopped celery
1 green pepper
1 onion

Marinade Sauce:
1 can of tomato soup
⅓ cup sugar
1 tsp. mustard
½ cup of salad oil
⅓ cup vinegar
1 tsp. Worcester sauce

To be prepared a day in advance.

Cook the carrots until barely soft, still firm. Layer in a casserole dish and pour marinate over. Refrigerate overnight.

ITALIAN GREEN PEPPERS

Serve with fried chicken, veal cutlets, or meatloaf.

½ cup onion, thinly sliced
2 cloves garlic, minced
2 tbsps sugar
4 - 5 large green peppers, cut into strips ¾" wide
1 tbsp. salad oil
2 cups stewed tomatoes
1 tsp. salt
½ tsp. basil
3 tbsps salad oil
dash pepper

Cook onion and garlic in 1 tbsp. oil until tender. Add tomatoes, sugar, and basil. Simmer for 20 minutes. Cook pepper strips in 2 tbsps. oil, turning frequently, till tender and still crisp. Lift from oil to serving dish. Sprinkle with salt and pepper. Pour over tomato sauce.
Serves five to six.

In 1996 a strange smell was permeating the basement of my parent's home. Father, Kerry, and I searched around the basement trying to determine the cause. We checked the freezer to ensure it hadn't come unplugged, and looked in cupboards. As we were about to give up I noticed a plastic grocery bag sitting behind the door against the wall next to the freezer. I peeked inside and found the source of the smell, a previously frozen turkey, with its juices spilling onto the cement floor. Father carried the bag out to the garbage. He said Mother had purchased the turkey the week before because it was on sale at the grocery store. She was only inches away from completing her mission to put it into the freezer. She must have put the bird down to lift the lid of the freezer, then became distracted by something, went to another part of the house, and forgot all about the turkey.

ZUCCHINI CASSEROLE

Given to Mother by her friend Joyce Shulz.

3 lbs. zucchini, cubed
4 eggs, well beaten
¼ cup melted margarine for sautéing
1 large onion, chopped fine
2 cups shredded cheddar cheese
3 cups breadcrumbs
¼ cup melted margarine
salt and pepper to taste

Sauté onion, mix with zucchini, eggs, and cheese and toss to coat. Put in 2 greased casserole dishes. Mix breadcrumbs and melted margarine, and sprinkle on top of zucchini mixture. Bake 45 to 60 minutes at 350° F. Each dish serves four.

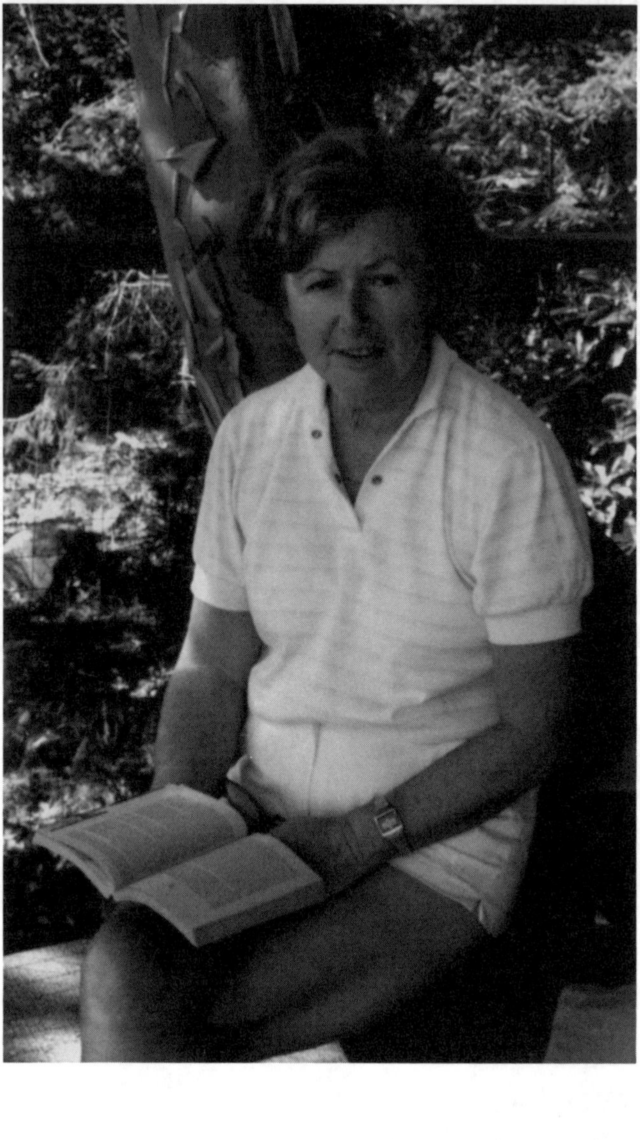

SEAFOOD AND FISH

STAGE 3: MILD COGNITIVE DECLINE

During Stage 3 of Alzheimer's Disease the symptoms the patient is exhibiting become more noticeable to others. The patient is in the early confusional stage and mild cognitive decline, and functioning at the skills level of a young adult. The person with Alzheimer's Disease will deny anything is wrong, but people around the patient become aware of the person's poor performance in carrying out common tasks, and word and name finding deficit becomes evident to others. Some patients are very skilled at disguising that anything is wrong. The patient may show symptoms of mild to moderate anxiety, and verbal outbursts, agitation, and tearfulness may become frequent. The patient may get lost when travelling to an unfamiliar location, unable to comprehend a map or road signs. The patient will read newspapers and books but retain little material.

Other symptoms may include:

- Difficulty remembering names when introduced to new people.
- Patient may have lost or misplaced an object of value.
- Patient suggests people are stealing things.

At this stage, the concentration deficit may be evident upon clinical testing.

DRIVING

A patient with Alzheimer's Disease isn't always incapable of driving. Mother was a careful driver, able to understand traffic lights and road signs. She never had an accident. We monitored her driving very carefully, and most of her destinations were within a few miles of my parent's home, and places that were well known to her for many years.

As the disease progresses and the patient shows signs of loss of orientation, judgment, and traffic flow, or when driving is recognized as dangerous, then access to the vehicle should be immediately removed. Signs that driving abilities are declining might include traffic violations or accidents on a person who previously had a clear record. Slow response times, taking too much time to reach a destination, or not reaching the destination at all, are indicators the patient needs to stop driving. A few patients will recognize their decreasing ability to operate the vehicle and stop driving on their own. More commonly the patient resists. Being unable to drive can be devastating and is a major loss of independence to the patient. It may be necessary to hide the keys, hide the vehicles, or modify the vehicle so that it can not be driven.

My father had devices installed in both vehicles which cut off power to the engine. Some Alzheimer's patients are smarter and sneakier than you give them credit for. They may be capable of picking up a guest's keys and driving off in their car, so make sure your guests keep their keys with them. When Mother received her driver's license renewal in the mail, my father managed to hide it before she saw it. A short time later we had a doctor's certificate forwarded to the motor vehicle licensing branch which cancelled her license and would prevent any attempt to renew it. For a few months, my mother would offer to drive and sometimes get behind the driver's seat first, but eventually she stopped asking to drive.

ALL IN ONE QUICHE

This recipe came from Mother's friend, Martha Watson, who still lives in Scotland.

1½ cups milk
½ cup biscuit mix
6 tsps. butter, at room temperature
3 eggs
1 cup diced fish or seafood
2 green onions, chopped
¼ pound mushrooms
1 cup grated sharp cheese
salt and pepper to taste

Preheat oven to 325° F. Mix milk, biscuit mix, butter, eggs, salt, and pepper and pour into well greased deep pie dish. Add seafood. Top with onions, mushrooms, and cheese. Bake at 325° F oven for 45 minutes to one hour, until golden brown. Let stand for 10 minutes before serving.

Mother would hide things away in strange places. We never knew where something would unexpectedly turn up. Once I found a chocolate bar in her jewelry box, but other times she'd hide chocolate bars, clothing, and kitchen utensils that would be unearthed months later.

AUNTY PASTO'S SEAFOOD LASAGNA

Your family and friends will ask for seconds.

8 lasagna noodles
1 cup onion, chopped
2 tbsps. butter
1 package (250 gram) cream cheese, softened
1½ cups creamed cottage cheese
1 egg, beaten
2 tsp. dried basil
2 cans cream of mushroom soup
⅓ cup milk
⅓ cup dry white wine
1 can (127 gram) crab meat
500 grams shrimp
¼ cup grated parmesan cheese
½ cup grated old cheddar cheese
½ tsp. salt
¼ tsp. pepper

Cook noodles in boiling salted water. Drain and place four noodles in 9" x 13" baking pan.

Preheat oven to 350° F. In saucepan, sauté onion in butter until soft. Remove from heat and let cool. Add cream cheese, cottage cheese, egg, basil, salt and pepper. Spread half the cream cheese mixture over noodles.

Combine soup, milk, and wine. Stir in crab meat and shrimp. Spoon half the mixture over cheese layer. Repeat all layers. Sprinkle with parmesan cheese. Bake uncovered at 350° F for 45 minutes. Sprinkle cheddar cheese over top and brown under broiler. Let stand 15 minutes before serving.

Serves eight to ten.

BAKED SALMON

Sliced lemons add color and zest.

6 lb. salmon
2 – 3 cups bread crumbs
4 tbsps. butter
1 small onion, minced
¼ tsp. rosemary
1 tsp. salt
⅛ tsp. pepper
½ tsp. thyme
1 tbsp. malt vinegar
1 cup celery, chopped
2 tbsps. grated cheese

Preheat oven to 450 degrees F. Melt butter in saucepan. Add onion and cook until onions are golden brown and tender. Add all ingredients and mix well. Stuff the fish. Use foil to line pan and let fish lie on celery leaves. Bake at 450 degrees F for 45 minutes.

> One day Mother arrived home from her hairdresser in Cloverdale, about a 12 mile round trip. The gas tank in the car had gone down significantly indicating she probably got disoriented on the way home, and had driven around for awhile before finding the correct way home.

BOSTON CLAM CHOWDER

Serve this is soup bowls made from sourdough bread.

2 lbs. clams in the shell
½ cup chopped bacon (optional)
¼ cup chopped onion
1 cup clam liquor and water
1 cup diced potatoes
2 cups milk
½ tsp. salt
dash pepper
parsley

Thaw clams, if necessary, shuck, and drain, saving the liquor. Chop. If using bacon, fry and lightly brown. Add onion and cook until tender. Add chopped clams, clam liquor, potatoes, and seasonings. Cook gently 15 minutes until potatoes are tender. Add milk and heat. Do not boil. Garnish with chopped parsley.

One day Mother arrived home and said she was driving the wrong way down a one-way street and people were honking at her. She was unable to tell us where this happened, but we guess within a couple of miles from home. She didn't seem at all concerned about the incident.

CHOPSTICK TUNA CASSEROLE

Quick and easy, this has always been one of my favorite meals. Serve with warm dinner rolls or toast.

1 can cream of mushroom soup
¼ cup water
3 oz. chow mein noodles
1 can (7 oz) tuna
1 cup sliced celery
½ cup toasted cashew nuts
¼ cup chopped onion
1 small can mandarin orange slices (optional)
dash of pepper

Preheat oven to 375° F . Combine soup and water. Add 1 cup noodles, tuna, celery, cashews, onion, pepper and toss lightly. Place in casserole dish in 375° F oven for 20 minutes. Garnish with mandarin orange sections. Serves four.

CLAMS IN WHITE WINE FOR TWO

Serve with French bread.

2 lbs. clams
½ cup parsley, finely chopped
6 tbsp. olive oil
1 garlic clove, finely chopped
½ cup dry white wine
juice of 1 lemon

Place clams in a shallow copper pan or flame proof casserole with parsley, olive oil, and garlic. Cover the pan tightly and steam for about 3 to 5 minutes, until clams open. Pour dry white wine into pan and simmer mixture for 1 minute. Squeeze the lemon juice over the clams and serve them hot from the pan.

CREOLE STYLE FISH

A low calorie meal that's great with warm crusty bread.

1 large green pepper, sliced thin
1½ cups chopped green onion
2 tbsps. butter or margarine
1 can (14 oz.) chopped tomatoes
1 can (7½ oz.) tomato sauce
½ tsp. thyme
1 bay leaf
1½ lbs. fish fillets (sole, cod, or halibut)
salt, pepper
3 cups hot cooked rice

Preheat oven to 375 ° F. Sauté green pepper and onion in butter till tender. Stir in tomatoes, sauce, one tsp. salt, ¼ tsp. pepper, thyme, and bay leaf. Simmer gently for 20 minutes. Remove bay leaf.

Arrange fish fillets in a lightly greased shallow baking pan. Season with salt and pepper. Spoon sauce over fillets. Bake in moderate oven, 375 ° F for 15 minutes or until fish flakes easily with a fork. Serve over rice.

In April, 1997 while her sister and brother-in-law from England were visiting, Mother backed the van out of the carport, completely oblivious that she had hit the side of the garage on the way out, damaging the van. My aunt and uncle had witnessed the accident, and after that didn't want to be in the vehicle if she was the driver, to the point of phoning Kerry and I to ask if we were available to drive them.

MOULES MARINIERE OR PROVENÇALE

Delicious and easy to prepare in less than thirty minutes.

3 tbsps. butter or margarine
1 clove garlic, minced or pressed
½ cup lightly packed minced parsley
1 small onion, chopped
1 cup dry white wine
⅛ tsp. pepper
about 30 live mussels in shells

In a large pot melt the butter over medium heat. Add onion and garlic, stirring occasionally till soft. Add wine, parsley, and pepper. Bring mixture to the boil. Add mussels, cover, and simmer gently until mussels have opened (about 5 to 8 minutes).

Throw away any mussels that do not open!

Moules Provençale

Prepare above recipe, but increase garlic to 3 cloves, minced or pressed. Cook onion, garlic, and ½ cup chopped celery in the butter until soft. Add 1 can (398 ml) whole tomatoes and their liquid and ⅛ tsp. cayenne. Simmer, covered, for 15 minutes. Then add wine, parsley, pepper and finally mussels, cooking as directed above.

> We wrote the B.C. Department of Motor Vehicles on June 27, 1997 in an attempt to get Mother's drivers license revoked. In typical government fashion, all they did was send a standard letter thanking us for warning them of an unsafe driver and didn't take any further action.

SALMON FILLETS WITH MANGO

Steamed rice completes this meal.

4 - 6 ounces of salmon fillets (650 grams)
3 tbsps. chopped green onions
3 tbsp. sherry
2 tbsp. lime juice
1 tbsp. soy sauce
1½ tsp. grated fresh ginger
1 garlic clove, finely chopped
2 tsps. vegetable oil
1 tsp. grated lime rind
1 ripe mango, peeled and sliced (or replace with papaya)

Preheat oven to 450° F . Place salmon skin side down in greased 13"x 9" baking dish. In small bowl whisk together remaining ingredients except mango. Pour over salmon. Bake uncovered at 450° F for 15 minutes or until salmon flakes easily when tested with a fork. Serve with mango wedges. Serves four.

> Mother's driver license renewal arrived in the mail in September, 1997 and was hidden by my Father.

SCALLOPED SALMON

Add flair and flavor to leftover salmon.

1½ cups cold cooked flaked salmon
1 cup thick white sauce
1 tbsp. chopped green pepper
¼ tsp. paprika
1 cup breadcrumbs

Preheat oven to 400 °F. Mix salmon, hot white sauce, green pepper. Add paprika. Put in greased baking dish. Sprinkle with breadcrumbs. Bake in hot oven 400° F till crumbs are brown.

White sauce:

2 tbsps. butter or margarine
2 tbsps. Flour
¼ tsp. Salt
dash pepper
1 cup milk

Melt butter or margarine in small saucepan. Stir in flour, salt, and pepper. Add milk. Cook and stir over medium heat till thickened and bubbly. Yield, one cup.

Through the help of an MLA in October, 1997, we managed to get the Department of Motor Vehicles to send a medical form that had to be filled out by a doctor to determine whether or not Mother was capable of driving. After perseverance on our part, the Acting Superintendent of Motor Vehicles cancelled her driver's license on November 18, 1997 – six weeks after the license had expired!

SEAFOOD CASSEROLE

Garnish with sliced olives and parsley to add zest to this succulent dish.

1½ lbs. haddock or cod
4 oz. peeled shrimp
4 oz. scallops
1 can (12 oz.) whole kernel yellow corn, drained
1 can (15 oz.) artichoke hearts, drained and quartered
1 small jar pimentos
½ cup flour
1 cup milk
1 tsp. Dijon mustard
1 tsp. lemon juice
¼ cup sour cream
¼ cup mayonnaise
⅓ cup white wine to thin sauce

Preheat oven to 375° F. Cut uncooked fish into 1 inch cubes. Combine the fish cubes, peeled shrimp and scallops in a large, fairly shallow 2 quart baking dish. Toss with the corn, artichoke hearts and pimento.

Melt butter in a medium sauce pan. Stir in the flour and let cook one minute. Gradually stir in milk, whisking to make a smooth, thick sauce after bringing it to a boil. Remove from heat and whisk in the mustard, lemon juice, sour cream and mayonnaise.

Adjust thickness of sauce with white wine as desired. Pour over seafood and vegetables while still very hot. Stir gently to coat. Bake for 20 minutes at 375° F or until the fish test done and sauce is bubbly. Serves six.

Note: If the sauce is hot when added to the raw seafood, 20 minutes oven time is adequate to cook it. Fresh seafood should be used.

SHRIMP CURRY

Fiery flavors borrowed from the East.

1½ cups fresh shrimp
¼ cup butter or margarine
1 large onion, chopped
3 tsps. flour
1 can beef bouillon
1 cup apple sauce
1½ tsp. curry
¼ tsp. salt
¼ tsp. ground ginger
dash cayenne
2½ tbsp. lemon juice
3 cups cooked rice

Melt butter or margarine. Add onion and fry for 5 minutes. Stir in flour, mixing for a minute. Add beef bouillon, apple sauce, curry, ginger, salt, cayenne, and lemon juice. Stir well. Add shrimp, and simmer 15 minutes. Serve over rice. Accompany with shredded coconut, chutney, bananas, and peanuts.

It became increasingly difficult to take Mother to the movies because she was unable to comprehend much of the show. Movies by Disney were a good choice. Comedies geared toward younger viewers were good because the subject matter was easy for her to understand.

SNOW CRAB CASSEROLE

Also known as Grey Cup Crab Casserole, Mother got this recipe from her friend Marguerite Leach, who'd serve this dish at football parties.

2 packages (6 oz. each) frozen Atlantic snow crab, thawed and drained
½ green pepper, sliced
¼ cup onion, finely chopped
3½ tbsps. butter
2 cups cooked rice
1 cup grated cheese
2 hard cooked eggs, sliced
1½ tbsps. flour
1½ cups milk
1½ tbsps. mayonnaise
¾ tsp. salt
⅛ tsp. pepper
½ cup dry bread crumbs

Preheat oven to 350° F . Sauté green pepper and onion in one tbsp. butter until soft. Place rice in a 2 quart casserole and layer with half the crab, cheese, egg slices, remaining crab, green pepper and onion. Melt 1½ tbsps. butter in a pan. Blend in flour, then milk. Cook and stir over low heat. Stir in mayonnaise, salt and pepper. Pour sauce over casserole ingredients, sprinkle with bread crumbs and dot with reaming one tbsp. butter cut into bits. Bake at 350° F 30 to 40 minutes.

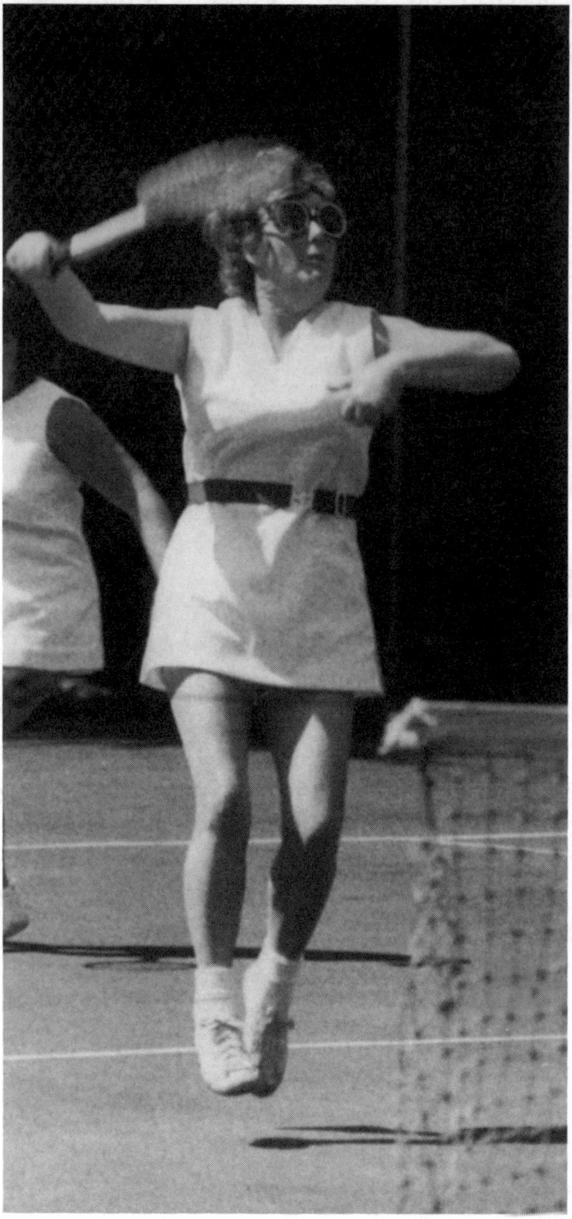

MEAT DISHES

STAGE 4: MODERATE COGNITIVE DECLINE

At Stage 4 of Alzheimer's Disease symptoms are very obvious. The patient has difficulty with complex tasks, and is functioning at the skills and ability level of an eight year old child to a teenager.

The patient becomes forgetful of personal history, has difficulty concentrating, and withdraws from challenging situations. The patient shows a decrease in ability to handle finances, go shopping, travel, and plan meals. The Alzheimer's patient is frequently unable to tell what time and date it is, and knowledge of current and recent events decreases. The patient may be unable to recognize familiar people or travel to familiar locations. Verbal outbursts, tearfulness, depression, and delusions may increase, but the patient may become less anxious and agitated in certain situations. Denial that anything is wrong becomes a strong defense mechanism.

AROMATIC BEEF STEW WITH GREEN BEANS AND CILANTRO

This savory stew can be frozen.

2 pounds boneless beef chuck
1 large onion, chopped
2 cans (796 ml) whole plum tomatoes, drained, chopped
1 tbsp. curry powder
1 tbsp. grated fresh ginger root
3 tbsps. fine chopped cilantro
3 tbsps. vegetable oil
1 tbsp. plus 1 tsp. all purpose flour
¾ cup water
2 garlic cloves, crushed
¾ pound green beans, trimmed and broken in 2 pieces
salt and fresh ground pepper

Preheat oven to 450° F. Trim excess fat from beef and cut into 1½ inch pieces. Heat oil in four quart heavy flameproof casserole. Brown meat in batches. Remove meat to a plate using a slotted spatula. Add onion to casserole and cook over low heat, stirring often until softened. Return meat to casserole reserving any juices on plate. Sprinkle with flour, tossing lightly to coat. Bake uncovered at 450° F, for five minutes, stirring once. Remove casserole and reduce oven temperature to 325° F. Pour juices from plate over beef and stir in tomatoes and 1¾ cups water or enough to barely cover beef. Add curry powder, garlic, ginger, salt, pepper and 2 tbsps. cilantro and bring to a boil, stirring frequently. Cover and bake about 1½ hours or until meat is tender. Stir occasionally. Cook green beans in boiling salted water until tender crisp. Drain and add to stew. Stir in remaining cilantro. Adjust seasoning if necessary. Serves six.

BARBECUED FLANK STEAK

Round up your family and friends and fire up the barbecue.

1 flank steak (about 1½ pounds or 750 grams)

Marinade:
½ cup soy sauce
2 tbsps. honey
2 green onions, chopped
¼ cup lemon juice
2 tbsps. peanut or olive oil

Place flank steak in shallow dish or pan. Combine marinade ingredients and pour over steak. Marinate overnight in the refrigerator, turning steak occasionally. Cook over hot coals for about five minutes on each side, brushing frequently with marinade. Carve steak diagonally across the grain into thins slices. Serves four to five.

Mother had her money in accounts with two different banking institutions. She would go to one bank and withdraw ten one hundred dollar bills, then go to the second bank to deposit the cash. One day she arrived home and told my father she wasn't sure if she had put the $1000 into the correct account. She had the deposit slip and it showed she had deposited the money into a bank account that wasn't hers. Father drove up to the bank immediately and got the mistake straightened out, and the money was transferred from the stranger's account back into Mother's account. After that Mother didn't show much interest in banking matters and Father arranged for a power of attorney and took over her financial transactions.

BEEF AND BROCCOLI - CHINESE STYLE

Serve this Oriental dish with rice or noodles.

1 lb. flank steak
¼ cup Soya sauce
1 tbsp. corn starch
1 tbsp. dry sherry
1 tsp. sugar
½ bunch broccoli
5 tbsp. vegetable oil
½ tsp. salt
½ cup onion, sliced

Slice beef finely across the grain in ¼ inch slices 2 inches long. Mix beef with Soya sauce, corn starch, sherry, and sugar and set aside. Cut broccoli tops in flowerets 2 inches long and ¼ inch thick. Pour 2 tbsps. oil in hot skillet over high heat. Add salt and broccoli and stir fry for 2 minutes. Remove and keep warm. Add remaining oil to skillet and sliced onion. Stir in beef mixture and stir fry 2 to 3 minutes or till done. Add broccoli and mix lightly.

I kept one of Mother's department store credit cards at my house so she wouldn't lose it. I would take her to the store to go shopping and when it came time to pay I would pull out the credit card and let her sign the slip, but I would take the credit card back. This gave her the independence to make purchases, while giving us peace of mind that the credit card would not be lost anywhere.

BEEF AND NOODLES SUPREME

Can be frozen and served later.

4 cups uncooked noodles
3½ cups chopped onions
2 tbsps. butter
2 lbs. ground beef
2 tsps. salt
½ tsp. pepper
3 eggs, well beaten
1 tsp. thyme
1 can cream of celery soup
1 can (14 oz) whole kernel corn
⅓ cup skim milk powder
1½ cups shredded cheddar cheese

Preheat oven to 350° F. Cook noodles in large amount of boiling salted water, adding butter to prevent boiling over. Sauté onions in butter, set aside. Brown meat in same pan. Drain off excess fat. Add onions, seasonings, soup, corn and milk powder, mix well. Alternate layers of noodles and meat mixture, ending with noodles. Top with cheese then beaten eggs. Bake uncovered 350° F for one hour. Serves ten to twelve.

One of Mother's favorite phrases was "I have nothing." She would go on further to say "I have no money. I have no clothes. I have no car. I have nothing." Father always put a small amount of money in Mother's purse. She was constantly misplacing her purse, so if it went missing for good, there wouldn't be a lot of money lost.

BEEF AND PEPPERS

Delicious served over hot rice or noodles.

2 tbsps. vegetable oil
1 medium red bell pepper, cut into thin strips
1 medium green pepper, cut into thin strips
1 medium onion, sliced thin
500 gr. flank steak, cut into thin strips
¼ cup dry red wine
1 can (796 ml) tomatoes with herbs and spices
1 tsp. dried oregano
½ tsp. dried thyme
1 tbsp. all purpose flour
2 tbsps. water
hot cooked noodles
salt and pepper to taste

Heat one tbsp. oil in large fry pan over medium heat. Sauté red and green peppers for about five minutes or until tender. Remove from pan and set aside. Add remaining one tbsp. oil to fry pan and heat. Add beef and onion. Stir fry until beef is cooked. Drain off liquid in fry pan. Add tomatoes and wine. Bring to a boil. Stir in peppers, oregano and thyme. Bring to a boil. Stir together flour and water. Pour into fry pan and cook until bubbling and thickened. Season to taste with salt and pepper. Serve over hot rice or noodles. Serves four.

BEEF BURGUNDY

Mother received this recipe from her friend Marguerite Leach.

2 - 5 lbs. top or bottom round steak
$^{1}/_{3}$ cup flour
2 tsp. salt
¼ tsp. pepper
6 tbsps. margarine
3 tbsps. brandy
3 medium carrots, sliced
3 medium onions, sliced
3 sprigs parsley (or dried)
2 bay leaves
dash of thyme
1 clove of garlic
3 cups dry red wine
3 slices of half cooked bacon
1 can (284 ml) sliced mushrooms
1 small can (156 ml) tomato paste

Cut meat into 1½ inch cubes. Combine flour, salt and pepper and coat each cube. Melt 4 tbsp. margarine in heavy pot and brown meat on all sides. Pour brandy over meat and set it aflame. In separate pan, melt 2 tbsp. margarine and sauté carrots and onions for five minutes. Add to meat, also add parsley, bay leaves, thyme and garlic, and stir. Add the red wine, enough to cover meat (the quantity depends on amount of meat used). Add mushrooms and tomato paste. Stir well. Cook 30 minutes longer.

Serve with wild rice and green peas for color.

BEEF PRIME RIB WITH YORKSHIRE PUDDING

Serve on a platter with puddings and roasted onions.

5½ - 6 lbs. prime rib roast of beef
3 tbsps. soft butter
¼ tsp. black pepper
8 - 10 small onions, peeled
3 garlic cloves, cut in slivers
1 tsp. coarse pickling salt
2 tsps. dried thyme leaves, crushed
olive oil

Preheat oven to 350° F. Rub olive oil over portions of meat not covered by fat. Place garlic clove slivers in various nooks and cavities in the roast. In a medium custard cup blend butter, salt, pepper and thyme. Rub over meat. Place meat, rib side down on rack in roasting pan. Place onions in pan. Roast 15 minutes per pound for rare, 20 minutes per pound for medium rare. Remove pan from oven. Place roast and onions on a preheated platter in a warm place for 25 minutes. Increase oven temperature to 425° F in preparation of the puddings.

Yorkshire Pudding:
2 large eggs, beaten
1 tbsp. beef drippings from roast
½ tsp. salt
1 cup milk
1 cup flour

Combine all ingredients in a bowl. Whisk or beat until smooth. Grease 12 muffin cups (use fat from roast if possible) and pour in batter. Bake for 25 to 30 minutes at 425° or until puffed and browned. Remove from muffin cups. Make a small slit in the bottom of each with a sharp knife. Use any remaining fat from roast to prepare gravy, if desired. Serves eight to ten.

CHICKEN AND PEACHES PIQUANT

Another recipe Mother got from her friend Marguerite Leach. Great served over a bed of rice.

2 whole skinned and boned chicken breasts
1 can (14 oz) sliced peaches
1½ tbsp. oil
1 large green pepper cut in squares
1½ tsp. seasoned salt
½ tsp. pepper
1 large onion, sliced
1 cup ketchup
2 tbsps. soy sauce

Cut chicken into thin strips. Sprinkle with salt and pepper. Sauté chicken in oil for two minutes, adding onion till it is tender. Drain peaches, reserving syrup. Blend ketchup and peach syrup with enough water to make two cups of liquid. Add soy sauce. Pour over chicken and simmer for 20 minutes. Cool and add peaches and green pepper. This recipe can be frozen.

CHICKEN RICE CASSEROLE

Great served with your favorite steamed vegetables.

3 lbs. chicken parts
1 cup brown rice
1 can cream of celery soup
1 can cream of mushroom soup
½ package dry onion soup

Mix rice, soups and water in oblong casserole. Lay chicken pieces on top, and shake onion mix over all. Bake covered in oven 350° F for 1½ to 2 hours till chicken is tender.

CLAY POT BEEF STEW

This is great served over wide egg noodles.

2 medium onions, sliced
3 lbs. stewing beef in 2" cubes
2 cloves garlic, minced
2 cups dry red wine
1 can consommé soup
½ cup water
1 bay leaf
¼ lb. mushrooms, sliced and sautéed
8 medium carrots, peeled and sliced
3 tbsps. flour
2 tbsps. parsley
salt and pepper to taste
parsley

Place onions in clay cooker which has been soaked in water for 10 minutes. Arrange meat over onions and cover. Place in cold oven, then turn heat to 400° F. Bake one hour. Add garlic, wine, consommé, seasonings, and bay leaf. Cover and cook for another hour. Add mushrooms and carrots. Cook another hour. Stew may be served as is or thickened by pouring liquid into saucepan and thicken with flour dissolved in water. Add meat to sauce. Sprinkle with parsley .
Serves six to eight.

One day Mother needed £5 for a college alumni magazine she wanted to subscribe to. When she left the house, Father followed her, and caught up with her half a mile away wandering in the parking lot of a shopping mall. She was looking for the currency exchange shop, but she hadn't brought any money with her to purchase the British pound. Father asked her how she planned to get the £5 and she said the clerk would just hand it over to her for no money.

COMPANY CHICKEN WINGS

Delicious served hot or cold. This is best served with a salad, but it can also be used as a starter.

2 lbs. chicken wings
2 - 3 tsp. sugar
½ - ¾ cup soy sauce
2 tsps. minced ginger
1 clove garlic, minced
¼ tsp. pepper
½ tsp. paprika
½ tsp. chili powder

Trim tips off wings. Sprinkle chicken wings with sugar and allow to sit at room temperature for 15 to 20 minutes. Place chicken wings on baking sheet. In a 2 cup measure or small bowl add soy sauce, ginger, garlic, pepper, paprika and chili powder. Stir to combine. Pour over chicken and allow to sit 30 minutes, turning occasionally to completely coat chicken with the soy mixture. Place in 350° F oven for 45 minutes to one hour or until done.

Mother became obsessed with gardening. Unable to tell the difference between a plant and a weed, she'd pull out strawberry plants and flowers. She decided to trim the ferns one week, and spent days hacking them to pieces. Fortunately, they're a resilient plant and the fronds grew back. In the backyard is a cobblestone path, surrounded by pebbles. Mother would spend hours picking up each stone, pulling out any dead pine needles below it, and put them into a bucket.

ISOBEL'S PAELLA

A popular Spanish meal that Mother enjoyed during the time she spent on the Costa Brava.

1 frying chicken, cut in serving pieces
2 tbsps. flour
¼ cup olive or salad oil
1½ cups raw rice
1 large onion, chopped
1 clove garlic, minced
1 small green pepper, chopped
1 pimiento, cut into thin strips
1 lb. fresh peas, shelled
8 oz. clam juice
1½ cups water
1 chicken bouillon cube
½ tsp. salt
¼ tsp. pepper
⅛ tsp. marjoram
2 cans (7½ oz. each) minced clams
1 lb. fresh raw shrimps, shelled and deveined
4 tomatoes, peeled and sliced

Preheat oven to 350° F. Coat chicken pieces with flour. Brown in oil then place in large casserole. Sauté rice, onion, garlic, green pepper, and pimiento in oil in frying pan, stirring often for 10 minutes or until rice is golden. Spoon over and around chicken in baking dish. Top with peas and tomatoes. Heat clam juice, water, bouillon cube salt, pepper, and marjoram in same pan until cube dissolves. Pour over mixture in casserole. Cover. Bake at 350° F for 30 minutes. Add clams and shrimp and cook for a further 20 minutes or until warmed through.

LEMON CHICKEN

A beautiful combination of flavors complements the chicken.

2 whole chicken breasts
2 cups dry white wine
juice of 1 large lemon
½ tsp. salt
¼ tsp. ground ginger
2 - 3 tbsps. cornstarch
2 garlic cloves, minced
2 tbsps. salad oil
1 large onion, cut in chunks
1 head broccoli, separated into flowerets with sliced stems

Take the chicken meat off the bone and slice into strips. Place in a shallow dish. Combine the wine, lemon juice, salt, ground ginger, and minced garlic and pour over chicken. Cover and refrigerate overnight. Heat the oil in a wok or large skillet. Remove the chicken strips from the marinade and add to the wok. Stir fry quickly until the chicken turns opaque. Remove to a plate. Add the onion and broccoli stems to the wok and stir fry 2 minutes. Add the flowerets and mix well. Pour in all the marinade but reserve ¼ cup. Stir and cover for 1 minute. Remove cover. Mix the cornstarch with remaining marinade and pour into the wok. Add chicken and stir fry just until thickened.

MANGO BEEF STIR-FRY

Pacific Rim fruits and spices enhance the beef.

2 tbsps. soy sauce
1 garlic clove, chopped fine
2 tbsps. vegetable oil
1 pound flank steak, sliced thin
2 green onions, chopped
1 tsp. fine grated ginger
pinch dried crushed hot red pepper
2 mangoes, sliced

Sauce:
¼ cup beef broth
2 tsp. cornstarch
1 tbsp. soy sauce
¼ tsp. salt

Combine soy sauce, ginger, garlic, and hot pepper. Pour over meat strips and toss to coat. Combine sauce ingredients and set aside. Heat wok over high heat for about one minute. Add oil and heat. Add beef and stir fry until browned, about three minutes. Add sauce mixture and bring to a boil. Add mangoes and green onions and heat through. Serves four.

Mother became fond of recounting a story that took place during World War Two. She said she'd gone to France to return some books and was accompanied by British soldiers. Her sister kept trying to tell her it never happened, and that she had not traveled to France during the war. My mother was very insistent that the story was true. Eventually Aunt Sukey acknowledged her sister must have been a spy and gave up trying to convince her she did not travel to France.

MEXICAN FESTIVE TAMALE PIE

Olé! Serve this at your next fiesta.

1 cup chopped onion
1 tbsp. margarine
2 cups seasoned tomato sauce
1 cup chopped olives
1 tbsp. sugar
3 tsp. chili powder
1 cup chopped green pepper
¾ lb. ground beef
1½ cups whole kernel corn
1 clove garlic, minced
1 tsp. salt
dash pepper

Cook onion and green pepper in hot oil until tender. Add meat and brown. Add all the other ingredients and simmer 20 to 25 minutes. Serves five to six.

Mother often recounted a story about the next door neighbor's daughter who had some friends over for lunch. Mother says she invited them to set up their table in our driveway to hold their party. It started off as four or five girls and as she continually retold the story over the following months, it became about one hundred party goers. Mother and the next door neighbor did not get along, so there is no way my mother would have invited the daughter onto her property. The driveway at my parent's house is not very long, and is very steep with a hard curve. It would be impossible to set up a table and chairs as they would tip over and slide down the driveway due to the steep slope. One hundred people would not be able to fit on the driveway, and even four or five people would be pulled downwards by gravity.

ORANGE GINGER CHICKEN

An interesting blend.

½ cup orange juice
2 tbsps. lemon juice
2 tbsps. soy sauce
2 tbsps. sherry
2 tsps. grated fresh ginger
½ tsp. vinegar
¼ tsp. sugar
2 whole boneless chicken breasts, halved

In shallow baking dish combine orange juice, lemon juice, soy sauce, sherry, ginger, vinegar, and sugar.. Place chicken in marinade and let stand for 10 to 15 minutes, turning frequently. Remove chicken from marinade, and reserve marinade. Broil chicken for another five minutes per side or until cooked, turning once and brushing with marinade. Serves four.

ORIENTAL BURGERS

Dress up your ordinary hamburgers with Eastern flair.

1 pound ground beef
2 tsps. grated fresh ginger
2 tsps. hoi sin sauce
1/8 tsp. freshly ground pepper
2 tsps. soy sauce
2 tsps. dry sherry
1 green onion, finely chopped

In bowl combine all ingredients and mix well. Shape meat mixture into four patties. cook in fry pan for about 12 minutes or until well done, turning once. Serves four.

ORIENTAL LAMB

A simple way to jazz up your lamb.

1 tbsp. vegetable oil
8 lamb chops, 1 inch thick
2 garlic cloves, crushed
1½ tbsps. minced fresh ginger
¼ cup apricot jam
3 tbsps. Soya sauce

Heat oil in fry pan just large enough to hold chops. Add chops and cook over medium high heat just until lightly browned, about three minutes per side. Remove chops. Reduce heat to low and add remaining ingredients to pan. Simmer, covered, for five minutes, stirring often. Return chops to fry pan. Cover and simmer for three to four minutes, turning once, until lamb is cooked to desired doneness. If the chops are 2 inches thick, add a few minutes to cook. Serve chops with sauce poured over top. Serves four.

OVEN STEWING STEAK

Superb flavor!

2 pounds stewing beef
1 package dried onion soup
1 can cream of mushroom soup
1 cup red wine
1 medium onion, chopped

Preheat oven to 350° F. Put beef into a casserole and add onion soup mix, cream of mushroom soup, red wine and onion. Cover tightly and bake in 350° F oven for two hours. Serves four.

PORK AND B.C. MUSHROOMS SAUTÉ

Combine different types of mushrooms for an interesting appearance.

¾ pound boneless pork loin or tenderloin, cut into strips
1 tbsp. vegetable oil
2 green onions, thinly sliced
1 pound B.C. mushrooms
1 tbsp. butter
1 tbsp. soy sauce
2 tsps. finely grated fresh ginger
pinch freshly ground pepper

Clean mushrooms slice and set aside. In a medium size fry pan heat the butter and oil over medium heat. Add pork and sauté until no longer pink. Add mushrooms, soy sauce, green onions and ginger root. Sauté for three to five minutes or until the mushrooms are tender. Season with pepper.

By July, 1997 Mother was showing many symptoms of Stage 6. She was unable to know her birthday or family birthdays. She didn't remember long-time friends, but upon meeting them she carried on a conversation as if she'd just seen them the day before. Mother was very good at covering up memory deficiencies and choosing her own topics of conversation. Her personal hygiene was still good, and she was still able to play bridge.

PORK CHOPS WITH ROSEMARY

Add color to this meal with julienne carrots and zucchini, and complete the meal with parmesan rice and a green salad.

½ cup all purpose flour
¼ tsp. pepper
1 tbsp. vegetable oil
4 single loin pork chops
1 cup chicken stock
¼ cup dry white wine
1 tbsp. white wine vinegar
1 green onion, sliced
1 tsp. dried rosemary
1 tbsp. butter
fresh ground pepper to taste

Combine flour and ¼ tsp. pepper. Lightly dredge pork chops in flour, shaking off excess. Heat oil in large heavy fry pan over high heat. Add pork chops and fry for about 10 minutes or until cooked, turning once. Place on platter and set aside. Add chicken broth, wine, vinegar, green onion and rosemary to fry pan, scraping bottom of pan to loosen any browned bits. Bring to a boil over medium-high heat and cook until slightly thickened, about three to four minutes. Return chops to fry pan and heat through. Transfer pork chops to platter. Swirl butter into sauce and season to taste with pepper. Spoon sauce over pork chops. Serves four.

SHEPHERD'S PIE

Sure to please most everyone.

4 tbsps. butter, divided
2 carrots, peeled and chopped
3 tbsps. flour
2 tsps. Worcestershire sauce
1 large onion, chopped
2 pounds lean ground beef
1 can beef broth
2 tbsps. ketchup
1½ pounds potatoes, cooked
1 egg, lightly beaten
¼ tsp. pepper
½ tsp. salt
milk, as needed
½ tsp. fine herbs (optional)

Preheat oven to 425° F. Melt two tbsps. butter in saucepan. Add onion and carrots. Sauté until onions are tender. Add beef and cook, stirring frequently, until browned. Stir in flour and cook for one minute. Gradually stir in broth. Bring to a boil, stirring constantly. Add Worcestershire sauce, ketchup, herbs, salt, and pepper. Reduce heat, cover, and simmer for fifteen minutes. Spoon meat mixture into shallow 12" x 8" baking dish. Mash potatoes. Beat in the remaining 2 tbsps butter and enough milk to give a smooth and fluffy consistency. Season to taste with salt and pepper. Spread mashed potatoes over meat. Brush top with egg and bake at 425° F for 30 to 40 minutes or until the topping is browned and meat is heated through. Serves four.

SWEET AND SOUR PORK OR HAM, HAWAIIAN STYLE

Serve this at your next luau. Aloha!

1 tbsp. oil or margarine
1 onion, chopped
2 cups cooked pork or ham, cubed
2 tsps. cornstarch
2 tbsps. brown sugar
½ tsp. cloves
½ tsp. ginger
½ tsp. nutmeg
3 tbsps. lemon juice
2 tbsps. soy sauce
1 cup water
dash of salt

Heat oil or margarine in heavy skillet, and brown onions over medium heat. Add meat, browning slowly. Combine cornstarch with brown sugar and seasonings. Add lemon juice, soy sauce and water. Gradually stir into pork mixture. Cook, stirring continually until mixture thickens and comes to a boil. Reduce heat and simmer about 20 minutes. Serves four.

> Mother became frustrated when trying to turn on the CD player to listen to music. A common task for most people to put in a CD and turn on the power, this was a situation beyond her ability.

TOP OF THE ROUND STEAK BARBECUE

Quick to prepare. Serve with baked potatoes and grilled vegetables.

2 pound steak

Sauce:
3 tbsps. salad oil
2 tbsps. parsley
1 tbsp. lemon juice
2 tsps. salt
¾ tsp. rosemary
½ tsp. pepper
2 cloves garlic, crushed

Tenderize steak ahead of time. Mix together all ingredients for sauce. Grill steak 5 inches from medium hot coals for 15 minutes for rare, turning once and brushing with oil mixture.

TURKEY CUTLETS WITH PAPAYA GINGER SAUCE

This dish serves up subtle hints of the Orient.

500 grams turkey breast cutlets
1 tbsp. vegetable oil
1 tbsp. butter or margarine
1 green onion, chopped
1 garlic clove, finely chopped
⅓ cup chicken broth
¼ cup ginger marmalade
1 tbsp. lime juice
1 small papaya, peeled and cut into slices 2½ inches long
salt
freshly ground pepper

If necessary, pound cutlets to an even thickness. Sprinkle lightly with salt and pepper.

In fry pan heat oil and butter over medium heat. Add cutlets and fry about four minutes or until cooked, turning once. Remove cutlets to platter and keep warm.

Add garlic to fry pan, sauté for about one minute. Add chicken broth and boil for about two minutes or until slightly reduced, stirring and scraping browned bits from bottom of pan. Drain any juices from turkey cutlets into fry pan. Stir in marmalade and lime juice. Simmer for one minute. Add papaya and green onion. Cook until papaya is heated through, about two minutes, stirring frequently. Spoon over cutlets. Serves four.

VEGETARIAN DISHES

STAGE 5: MODERATELY SEVERE COGNITIVE DECLINE

In Stage 5 of Alzheimer's Disease the patient is at a moderately severe cognitive decline and early dementia. The patient functions at the level of a five to seven year old child and can no longer survive without some assistance. At this stage the patient may still retain facts about themselves and others, and still remember their name, and the names of their spouse and children.

The Alzheimer's patient encounters difficulty with numbers and becomes disoriented to time. They may be unable to recall their address, telephone number, and the names of relatives and friends. The patient may have difficulty choosing proper clothing to wear. This could mean dressing in summer attire during a winter storm, or putting on too many clothes for a hot day. The patient may begin layering clothing at this stage, putting on several items. It was not unusual for my mother to put on several pairs of underpants, pantyhose, socks, a couple of slips, a couple of dresses, or several shirts or sweaters.

Other symptoms might be:

- An increase in depression, suspiciousness and paranoia.
- Delusions that people are stealing their things.
- Fear of being left alone.
- May begin wandering away from caregiver or home.
- May begin to show sleep disturbance.
- Suffering delusions that this is not their house.

CRESCENT BEACH GOLF COURSE BEANS

You don't have to be a golfer to enjoy this dish.

½ cup minced onions
2 cloves garlic
1 tbsp. brown sugar
1 tsp. dry mustard
½ tsp. oregano
pinch of ginger
¼ cup ketchup
2 tbsps. vinegar
1 can (15 oz) kidney beans
1 can (15 oz) Boston beans
1 can (15 oz) Lima beans, drained

Fry onions and garlic. Add remaining ingredients and cook slowly for 20 minutes. Stir in beans. Put in bean crock and bake 30 to 40 minutes in 350°F oven.

The Non-Vegetarian Version:

Fry ½ pound of cut bacon with the onion and garlic. Reserve several strips of bacon to lay over the beans before cooking in the oven.

Mother didn't show any sleep difficulties or awaken in the night to wander. But she began to sleep a lot more, often going to bed early in the evening, shortly after eating dinner, and not waking up until eight or nine o'clock the following morning. Sometimes she would nap again later in the morning or the afternoon. Father was concerned she was sleeping so much, but the experts told us this was not unusual. In fact we were lucky. It is more common for Alzheimer's patients to have difficulty sleeping and get up several times during the night.

FALL HARVEST PASTA

A colorful medley of vegetables.

350 grams spaghetti
3 tbsps. vegetable oil
2 cups sliced mushrooms
1 small onion, chopped
2 garlic cloves, finely chopped
2 cups diced tomatoes
¼ cup grated Parmesan cheese
3 tbsps. butter
2 cups broccoli flowerets
1 small red bell pepper, cut in thin strips
¼ cup chopped parsley
2 tbsps. chopped fresh basil
salt and freshly ground pepper
grated Parmesan cheese

Cook spaghetti in large amount of boiling salted water until tender. Drain and keep warm. While pasta is cooking, heat butter and oil in large fry pan. Add broccoli, mushrooms, red pepper, onion and garlic to fry pan. Sauté until vegetables are tender crisp, about two to three minutes. Add tomatoes, parsley and basil. Cook about two minutes or until hot, stirring occasionally. Spoon vegetable mixture and ¼ cup Parmesan cheese over hot spaghetti. Toss well. Add salt and pepper to taste. Sprinkle each serving with Parmesan cheese. Serves four.

Mother had her own computer set up so that when she turned it on it went directly to a game of bridge. She'd spend hours playing bridge on the computer. She began arguing with it and telling us about the cheating bitches in her bridge game. One day she tried to pull the wires out of the back of the computer, intent on getting rid of the cheating bitches.

LINGUINI WITH B.C. MUSHROOMS AND PEAS

Dress up your linguini with color and flavor.

3 tbsps. butter or margarine
3 cups hot cooked linguini
1 cup frozen peas, cooked and drained
½ tsp. salt
375 grams B.C. mushrooms, sliced
½ cup half & half cream
½ cup grated Parmesan cheese
1 tsp. grated lemon peel
coarsely ground pepper

In a 10 inch skillet, over medium heat, melt butter and cook mushrooms until tender and liquid is evaporated, stirring occasionally. Add linguini, cream, peas, cheese, lemon peel, and salt. Toss to coat well. Heat through, stirring occasionally. Serve with coarsely ground pepper. Serves five.

Mother planted a pine needle garden. She gathered some pine needles, stuck them into the ground, got a watering can and watered them, and waited for them to grow.

OLIVE SWISS CHEESE PIE

A savory combination of cheeses and vegetables.

½ pound mushrooms, coarsely chopped
1¼ cups pitted olives, chopped
3 tbsps. butter or margarine
¼ cup dry breadcrumbs
½ cup green onions, chopped
1½ cups grated Swiss cheese
1 cup cottage cheese
3 eggs
½ tsp. thyme
¾ cup parsley, finely chopped

Preheat oven to 375° F. Sauté mushrooms and ¾ cup olives in butter till moist and coated (20 seconds). Stir in bread crumbs. Spoon into 9" pie plate and press evenly against bottom and sides. Sprinkle green onions, grated cheese and ½ cup olives into the shell. In blender, process cottage cheese, eggs, and thyme until smooth. Pour into pie shell. Bake at 375° F for 25 to 30 minutes or until a knife inserted in center comes out dry. Cover loosely with foil if it starts to get too brown. Serves six.

> One day I took Mother to McDonald's for a McFlurry treat. She saved the container the ice cream came in, and later filled it with water to carry to various parts of the garden to water the plants.

ORANGE RICE

A zesty kick to an old staple.

¼ cup butter or margarine
1 cup celery, diced
3 tbsps. chopped onions
2 tbsps. shredded orange peel
½ tsp. salt
¾ cup orange juice
¾ cup water
$1^1/3$ cups cooked rice

Over medium heat, melt butter in a skillet. Add celery, onion, and orange peel. Cook till celery and onion are tender but not brown. Add salt, orange juice, and water. Bring to a boil, then turn off heat. Stir in rice. Cover and let stand 7 minutes. Serves four to five.

When Mother was getting ready to play tennis, she would get dressed in pantyhose and a formal dress and announce she was ready to play a game. Even though she was in the wrong clothing, she would still remember to put on tennis shoes.

SPAGHETTI WITH ASPARAGUS AND MUSHROOMS

Spicy, colorful, and tasty.

2 tbsps. unsalted margarine
1 tbsp. vegetable oil
2 garlic cloves, finely chopped
750 gram asparagus, cut into 1 inch pieces
2 cups mushrooms, sliced
1 tbsp. chopped fresh basil
1 tbsp. chopped fresh oregano
1 tsp. chopped fresh rosemary
4 large plum tomatoes, diced
hot cooked spaghetti
grated Parmesan cheese
salt and freshly ground pepper to taste

Heat butter and oil in large heavy fry pan over medium high heat. Add garlic, asparagus, mushrooms, fresh herbs and cook until asparagus is tender crisp, about five minutes, stirring frequently. Stir in tomatoes. Season with salt and pepper. Remove from heat and add to hot cooked pasta. Toss. Sprinkle with Parmesan cheese. Serves four to five.

VEGETARIAN LASAGNA

A satisfying meal that will bring your guests back for seconds.

2 tbsps. oil
1 cup onions, sliced
½ cup diced carrots
½ cup diced celery
¼ tsp. garlic powder
1½ tsp. oregano
¼ tsp. celery seed
1 tsp. thyme
1½ tsp. ground rosemary
1½ tsp. basil
1 tsp. chili powder
1½ tsp. salt
2 cups tomato paste
1 tbsp. honey
2 cups water
8 oz cheddar cheese
8 oz mozzarella cheese
1 pound cottage cheese

Heat oil in a heavy skillet. Add onions and sauté for 5 minutes. Add carrots, celery, and garlic powder and sauté for 5 minutes. Add oregano, celery seed, thyme, rosemary, basil, chili powder, and salt and sauté one minute. Stir in tomato paste, honey, and water. Bring to a boil. Reduce heat and simmer one hour.

Cook 15 lasagna noodles according to package instructions. Preheat oven to 350° F.

Cover bottom of pan sparsely with sauce. Add a layer of noodles, cottage cheese, cheddar cheese and sauce. Repeat layers ending with mozzarella cheese and a little sauce on top. Bake at 350° F for an hour.

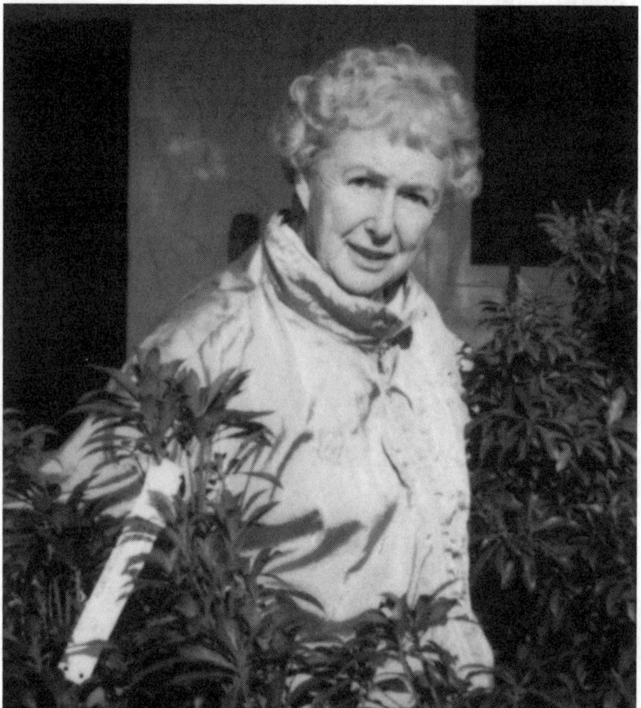

DESSERTS

STAGE 6: SEVERE COGNITIVE DECLINE

In Stage 6 the Alzheimer's Disease patient exhibits symptoms of severe cognitive decline and middle dementia. The patient is functioning at the skills level of a two to five year old child.

The patient can not carry a thought long enough to determine a course of action, and is often unaware of their surroundings, the year, season, and time. Knowledge of past life becomes sketchy and they are unaware of recent events and experiences in their lives. The patient is still able to distinguish familiar from unfamiliar persons in their environment, and able to recognize their own name, but they may forget the name of the person they are dependent on for survival. The patient will require some assistance with activities required for daily living, such as needing help to put on clothes. The patient may develop a fear of bathing and will require assistance bathing or being reminded when to bathe. Their ability to use the toilet decreases and the patient may become incontinent. The patient doesn't want to change their clothing and may sleep in their clothes, and wear the same items for several days.

Other symptoms consistent with Stage 6 are:

- Anxiety and obsessive symptoms.
- Suspiciousness and delusional behavior.
- Pattern of wandering.
- Fear of being alone.
- Tearfulness, outbursts, and depression related to comprehension and communication deficits.

BAKED CUSTARD

Easy to make and delicious!

½ cup flour
1 cup sugar
2 cups milk
½ cup melted butter
1 cup flaked coconut
4 eggs

Preheat oven to 350° F. Place all ingredients in a blender and mix for one minute. Place in 9" Pyrex pie plate and put in oven for one hour at 350° F.

I accompanied Mother on a trip to England in January, 1998 to visit her brother and sister. We had to take a train from London to her brother's town in Northern England. She was convinced that her brother lived in the south of England, and spent the two hour train ride hostile towards me because I had her on a train travelling in the wrong direction.

BRANDIED PUMPKIN CHEESECAKE

Serve this at Thanksgiving or Christmas as an alternative to pumpkin pie.

Crust:
1½ cups graham cracker crumbs
½ cup butter or margarine, melted
¼ cup sugar

Filling:
2 packages (250 gram) cream cheese
1 package (125 gram) cream cheese
1 cup sugar
4 medium eggs
1 can (14 oz.) pumpkin
2½ tsp. ginger
1 tbsp. cinnamon
½ tsp. nutmeg
¼ tsp. cloves
⅓ cup brandy
whipped cream
preserved ginger

For crust combine crumbs, sugar and butter in a bowl and mix well. Press crumb mixture firmly into bottom of 10" spring form pan and 2 inches up the sides. Bake in 350° F oven for 10 minutes.

For filling beat together cream cheese and sugar until light and fluffy. Add eggs one at a time, beating well after each addition until smooth and creamy. Add pumpkin, ginger, cinnamon, nutmeg, cloves, and brandy and mix until well blended. Pour cheese mixture into crust and bake in slow oven, 325° F for 50 to 60 minutes, or until well risen. Turn off heat and let cheesecake cool in oven. When cold, decorate top with whipped cream and sliced ginger.

CHRISTMAS DAY DESSERT

Delicious and fast!

1½ cups mincemeat
3 tbsps. brown sugar
6 tbsps. orange or lemon juice
½ cup pecans
¼ cup water
brandy (optional)

Heat all ingredients. Remove from heat and add brandy to taste, if desired. Pour over ice cream.

CRUMB TOPPED RHUBARB AND APPLES

Sweet and tart, serve with ice cream.

5 cups sliced rhubarb
1 cup brown sugar, divided
5 tbsps. all purpose flour, divided
¾ cup quick cooking oats
4 cups apples, peeled and sliced into ½" wedges
1½ tsps. ground cinnamon
⅓ cup cold butter

Combine rhubarb, apples, ⅔ cup sugar, 2 tbsps. flour, and cinnamon in four quart (four liter) microwavable casserole. In bowl combine remaining sugar and flour, and oats until well blended. Cut in butter until crumbly. Sprinkle over fruit. Microwave at HIGH for 15 minutes or until rhubarb is tender. Let stand for five minutes. Serves six.

> Unable to tell the difference between right and wrong, Mother took to poking people in the back with kitchen knives thinking it was a joke.

ORANGE FLUFF

This dessert makes you feel like you're floating on a cloud.

2½ cups small marshmallows
½ cup frozen orange juice
½ pint cream, whipped
¼ cup melted butter or margarine
¾ cup fine vanilla wafer crumbs
¼ cup finely chopped nuts

Line the bottom of a loaf pan with a crumb crust made by combining nuts, crumbs, and melted butter. Press firmly into the bottom of the pan. Heat marshmallows and juice over low heat till melted. Cool thoroughly. Fold in whipped cream. Pile into crumb crust and chill until firm.

Wandering began to be a problem. Mother would sneak out of the house and go for a walk. Sometimes a simple walk up and down the street to look at the flowers of neighboring houses. She frequently walked to the library, borrowing two or three books per week. She went through the motions of reading the books, but we doubted she was retaining any information. A walk to the library, around the corner and a block away, eventually confused her.

PARFAIT DESSERT

Choose your favorite fruit.

1 package (3 oz) fruit flavored Jell-O powder
1½ cups hot water or hot juice
1 pint ice cream
1½ cups sliced fruit, fresh or canned
1 tbsp. lemon juice

Dissolve Jell-O in hot water or juice. Stir in ice cream by spoonfuls until melted. Chill until thickened but not set. Fold in fruit and lemon juice. Chill in bowl or individual dishes.

PECAN PIE

You need a sweet tooth for this pie! Serve with ice cream or whipped cream.

9" unbaked pie shell
3 eggs, lightly beaten
1 cup corn syrup
1 cup brown sugar
1 cup chopped pecans
2 tbsps. melted butter
1 tsp. vanilla
$^{1}/_{8}$ tsp. salt
10 - 20 whole pecans for topping

Preheat oven to 375° F. Combine eggs, corn syrup, brown sugar, chopped pecans, butter, vanilla and salt in bowl, mixing well. Pour into pie shell. Decorate top with whole pecans. Bake at 375° F for 45 to 60 minutes, until middle of pie doesn't jiggle. Cool well before serving. Serves six to eight.

PINEAPPLE COCONUT DELIGHT

Memories of a Hawaiian vacation.

1 can (20 oz) pineapple tidbits
2½ cups miniature marshmallows
¼ cup well drained maraschino cherries, cut in quarters
1 cup whipping cream
$^{1}/_{3}$ cup shredded coconut

Drain pineapple reserving ½ cup syrup. Combine pineapple, marshmallows, cherries and ½ cup syrup. Let stand for one hour stirring occasionally. Beat cream till stiff and fold into pineapple mixture along with coconut.

It became increasingly difficult to get Mother to bathe. We tried coaxing and fooling her. We got bathtub accessories, and bubble bath beads that she liked. One evening my parents dropped over after being outside for awhile. My mother was cold and I suggested a bath would warm her up. She agreed it would be lovely, but didn't think she should take a bath at my house. I told her it was fine, ran a tub for her, dumped in a lot of bubble bath and washcloths and left her alone. When she was finished bathing she came back downstairs wearing her shoes, pantyhose, shirt, and her coat, but no pants. I asked her where her pants were and she said she didn't know, couldn't find them, and wasn't concerned about being half-dressed. I went back to the bathroom with her and the pants were sitting on the counter. I pointed them out to her and left her alone to put them on. When she came back downstairs, she was fully dressed.

PINEAPPLE FLUFF DESSERT

Prepare this hours before serving. Fluffy and silky, it's worth the wait.

2½ cup vanilla wafer crumbs
1 cup butter or margarine, divided
1½ cups sifted sugar
2 eggs
1 can (398 ml) crushed pineapple, drained
½ pint whipping cream, whipped

1st layer:
Combine 2 cups vanilla wafer crumbs and ½ cup melted butter or margarine. Place in pan or baking cups. Pat down firmly and bake in slow oven 300°F for 15 minutes. Cool.

2nd layer:
Beat with electric mixer ½ cup softened butter or margarine, sugar, and two eggs until light and fluffy. Spread over first layer.

3rd layer:
Combine can pineapple and whipped cream and place over second layer. Sprinkle remaining ½ cup crumbs over top. Refrigerate for several hours or overnight.

One day Mother walked to a stranger's house and knocked on the door. When a woman answered the door she asked to see Cheryl. The woman told her she had the wrong house, no one named Cheryl lived there. We have no idea whose house she went to. She told me about it later in great detail. I decided the easiest way to deal with it was to tell her that I had moved, and she was quite accepting of that explanation.

QUICK AND FLASHY DESSERT

Short on time? Try this tangy treat.

½ pound green seedless grapes
$^2/_3$ cup light sour cream
3 tbsps brown sugar
1 tsp. grated lemon peel

Blend by hand sour cream with brown sugar and grated orange peel. Toss in grapes and mix till coated. Spoon into wine glasses and chill in refrigerator.

VIENNESE TORTE

A wonderful dish for parties.

½ cup butter or margarine
½ tsp. salt
1 cup flour
½ cup apricot or plum jam

Filling:
3 tbsps. butter
6 eggs, separated
1¼ cups sugar
½ pound grated nuts

Cut butter into flour and salt till crumbly. Put into 10" spring form pan, covering bottom and ¼ inch on sides. Bake in 350° F oven for 15 minutes. Spread cake with jam. Cream butter and sugar together. Beat egg yolks and add to butter mixture till well blended. Gradually add nuts. Beat egg whites till stiff and fold into nut filling. Pour over jam. Bake at 325° F 30 to 40 minutes till firm. Some ovens could take up to an hour. Cake should not jiggle when shaken gently. Serves 12.

CAKES AND SQUARES

STAGE 7: VERY SEVERE COGNITIVE DECLINE

As the Alzheimer's Disease patient enters into the final stages of the disease, they are now in a very severe cognitive decline, and late dementia. At this point the patient is functioning at the skills ability of a 15 month old child, digressing to the level of a four week old baby.

The vocabulary of the patient becomes limited, declining to single words, until eventually all verbal abilities are lost. As a result the patient can't communicate any needs, or if they are in pain or discomfort. The brain is no longer able to tell the body what to do, and the patient loses basic psychomotor skills such as the ability to walk and sit. The patient is often off in their own little world, and unable to recognize familiar persons. In Stage 7 the patient becomes incontinent, and loses the ability to smile and hold their head up.

ALMOND SLICE

½ cup soft butter
1 tsp. almond flavoring
1 cup flour
1 cup white sugar
1 egg
¼ cup sliced almonds, or more to taste

Preheat oven to 375° F. Blend, by hand, butter, almond flavoring, sugar and egg. Add flour. Sprinkle with sliced almonds. Put in an 8" x 8" dish and place in oven at 375° F for 20 to 25 minutes.

During January, 1998 Father toured some intermediate care institutions and gave his three choices to the local case manager of the Continuing Care Division of the Ministry of Health and Ministry Responsible for Seniors. Waiting lists were one to four years.

BACARDI RUM CAKE

A superb combination of flavors.

1 cup chopped pecans
1 package (3¾ oz) Jell-O Vanilla instant pudding
½ cup cooking oil
1 package (500 gram) cake mix
½ cup cold water
4 eggs
½ cup rum

Glaze:
¼ lb. butter
1 cup granulated sugar
¼ cup water
½ cup rum

Preheat oven to 325° F. Grease and flour 10" tube pan. Sprinkle nuts over bottom of pan. Mix all cake ingredients together. Pour batter over nuts. Bake 1 hour. Cool. Invert on serving plate. Use fork to prink holes on top.

Glaze:
Melt butter in saucepan. Stir in water and sugar. Boil for 5 minutes, stirring constantly. Remove from heat and stir in rum.

Drizzle and smooth glaze evenly over top and sides. Allow cake to absorb glaze. Repeat till glaze is used up.

BROKEN GLASS CAKE

Colorful and delicious.

Crust:
1 cup graham wafer crumbs
1/3 cup sugar
1/3 cup butter
1 tsp. cinnamon

Combine crust ingredients and press into 13" x 9" pan. Chill.

Filling:
1 package (3 oz) strawberry or raspberry Jell-O
1 package (3 oz) lime Jell-O
1 package (3 oz) lemon Jell-O
½ pint whipping cream
½ cup sugar
1 envelope unflavored gelatin
½ cup cold water
½ cup hot water
¼ cup pineapple juice

Dissolve each Jell-O powder in 1½ cups hot water. Pour into separate pans and chill. Whip cream and sugar. Soften gelatin in ½ cup cold water and dissolve in hot water. Add pineapple juice. Mix into whipped cream.

Cut Jell-O into cubes. Add combined gelatin and whipped cream mixture to cubes. Pour into chilled crust. Chill. Serves twelve.

> In February, 1998 their doctor advised the downside to improved alertness from the Galantamine meant greater sensitivity to surrounding events which would account for frustrations and verbal outbursts.

BUTTER TART FILLING

A pleasing concoction that melts in your mouth.

½ cup Sultana raisins
2 tbsps. butter
½ cup white sugar
1 egg
1½ tsps. vanilla
boiling water

Preheat oven to 350° F. Pour boiling water over raisins, then drain. Mix in butter and add other ingredients. Bake at 350° F in 12 tart shells for 25 minutes.

Between March 1 to May 6, 1998 Mother had almost no person name recognition and rapidly deteriorating object name recognition. Declining logic and unable to separate the names or uses of items such as scissors, toothbrush, or garden tools. Layering of clothing was common, and she had to be coaxed to remove dirty underwear or take them off when going to bed. She had to be convinced and reminded to use a toothbrush or take a bath. She was highly impatient watching TV, movies, concerts, or observing traffic patterns. She was no longer able to play bridge. There were more hallucinations and she thought people were out to get her. She became more selective on foods and wouldn't eat salads, but liked soups and ice cream.

CARROT CAKE

Mother got this recipe from her friend Kay Todd.

2 cups flour
2 cups white sugar
1 tsp. cinnamon
4 eggs
3 cups grated carrots
½ tsp. salt
2 tsp. baking soda
1 tsp. allspice
1 cup corn oil

Mix dried ingredients. Add oil and stir in eggs, one at a time. Beat well after each egg. Add carrots. Pour into greased 13" x 8" pan. Bake at 350° F for 40 to 60 minutes.

Icing:
2 cups icing sugar
1 tsp. vanilla
¼ cup chopped walnuts
4 oz. cream cheese
¼ cup butter

Mix sifted icing sugar, cream cheese, vanilla and butter until fluffy. Spread on cake and sprinkle walnuts on icing.

Optional: Decorate with border of sugar frosting or whipped cream.

Alternative: Add 1 can crushed pineapple and ½ cup currants. Reduce carrots to two cups.

DOUBLE CHOCOLATE CAKE

An easy recipe for chocoholics.

1 package (2 layer size) Devil's Food chocolate cake mix
1 package (4 serving size) instant chocolate pudding mix
1½ tsps. cinnamon
½ tsp. cloves
1 cup sour cream
½ cup salad oil
½ cup warm water
4 eggs
1 6 oz package semi-sweet chocolate chips

Combine all ingredients except chocolate chips in large mixer bowl. Blend, then beat four minutes at medium speed on electric mixer. Fold in chocolate chips. Turn into greased and floured 10 inch Bundt pan. Bake according to directions on the cake mix.

In July, 1998 Mother began weekend visits to the V.O.N. Family Respite Centre in Vancouver. She went every couple of weeks, and it was a hotel-like atmosphere with many recreational activities to keep the patients busy during their stay. By August, 1998 Mother had no short-term memory and most of the long-term memory had also disappeared. She had no recollection of college, classmates, bridesmaids, and other people who had been part of her life. She had no realization of where her brother and sister lived and knew little about who they were, even though she spoke with them by phone every couple of weeks. She referred to everyone as "friends", even family members, as she no longer remembered names. There were bouts of inappropriate physical behavior. She tried to push my Aunt Margaret down a flight of stairs, and jokingly jabbed a knife into people's backs.

LEMON BREAD

The tangy lemon topping is the final touch.

6 tbsps. margarine or butter
1 cup white sugar
2 eggs, beaten
¼ tsp. salt
1 lemon rind, grated
1½ cups flour
2 tsps. baking powder
½ cup milk

Topping: Juice of 1 lemon, ½ cup sugar

Preheat oven to 350° F. Cream butter and sugar and add eggs. Sift dry ingredients and add to creamed mixture alternately with milk. Add lemon rind. Pour into greased loaf pan and bake in 350° F oven for 45 to 50 minutes or until it tests done. Mix topping and pour over loaf. Cook 5 minutes longer.

Alternative topping:
Mix 2 cups icing sugar with ⅓ cup lemon juice. After removing cake from oven, immediately make holes all over cake with large fork. Dribble icing over top of cake.

LEMON CAKE

Mother got this recipe from her friend Jean who was part of her weekly bridge club.

1 box yellow or white double cake mix
1 package (3 oz) lemon or pineapple Jell-O
¾ cup cold water
¾ cup salad oil
4 eggs
1 tsp. lemon or lemon flavoring

Use two 9 inch pans or 13" x 9" pan. Put cake mix and powder into bowl, add water, oil, and eggs. Beat 4 minutes then add lemon. Pour into cake pan and bake as instructed on the package.

NANAIMO BARS

This heavenly square will be gobbled down fast. Freezes well.

Crust:
½ cup butter, softened
¼ cup granulated sugar
5 tbsp. cocoa
1 tsp. vanilla
1 egg
2 cups graham wafer crumbs
1 cup coconut
½ cup chopped walnuts

Special Icing:
¼ cup butter
3 tbsps. milk
2 tbsp. vanilla custard powder
2 cups icing sugar

Top Layer:
4 squares semi-sweet chocolate
1 tbsp. butter

Place butter, sugar, cocoa, vanilla, and egg in bowl. Set bowl in pan of boiling water. Stir well till butter has melted and mixture resembles custard. Combine crumbs, coconut, and walnuts, mixing well. Add to cooked mixture. Pack evenly into 9" square pan.

Cream butter. Combine milk and custard powder and add to butter. Blend in icing sugar. Spread over cooled base. Let stand at least 15 minutes to harden.

Once custard has cooled, melt chocolate squares with butter in microwave oven or in a dish placed in boiling water. Spread over custard icing. When set, cut into bars.

PAVLOVA

Fill with your favorite fruit and whipping cream.

3 egg whites
1 tsp. vinegar
1 tsp. almond flavor
¾ cup berry sugar
1 tsp. corn starch
1 large brown paper bag

Preheat oven to 275° F. Beat egg whites until stiff for five minute in food processor and then add other ingredients. Mark a nine inch circle on the paper bag and place the meringue in the centre, forming a bird's nest.

Cook in a cool oven for an hour at 275° F. At the end of the hour, turn the heat off and open door to allow the meringue to dry out.

On August 23, 1998 Mother suffered a stroke while at the VON Family Respite Centre. She was transferred to Vancouver General Hospital for tests, and several days later transferred to Peace Arch Hospital in White Rock, closer to home. She now lives in the Extended Care Unit of the hospital. Two months after suffering the stroke, Mother discontinued the Galantamine. Mother is confined to a wheelchair and has limited use of her right arm and leg. Her speech is limited, but at times she is able to put together sentences. She undergoes physiotherapy for her arm and leg, but due to the Alzheimer's doesn't understand to do the exercises. She appears content in her new home and enjoys the activities and company of the other patients. One of the family is with her every day to assist her with lunch and dinner or to accompany her on the outings offered to the patients.

SPANISH ALMOND CAKE

Memories of Madrid.

6 large eggs, separated
¾ cup sugar
1 tsp. almond extract
2 cups ground almonds
2 cups whipping cream
½ tsp. sugar
2 tbsps. Amaretto liqueur
¼ cup toasted slivered almonds
pinch of salt

Preheat oven to 350° F. Butter a 10½" x 15½" jelly roll pan and line with wax paper. Butter again and coat with flour, tapping out the excess. Beat egg yolks with sugar until mixture thickens forming a ribbon which leaves a trail when beaters are lifted up. Add almond extract and ground almonds.

Beat egg whites with a pinch of salt until satiny peaks form. Mix a little beaten egg white into the yolk mixture, then fold remainder of the egg white in with a large spatula. Pour batter into the prepared pan and smooth it out.

Bake at 350° F for 20 minutes or until cake pulls away from the sides of the pan. Cool for a few minutes, then invert pan onto a piece of paper sprinkled with sugar. Peel off the wax paper and leave cake to become cold.

To Assemble:

Divide cake into two equal pieces. Place one piece on a square or rectangular serving platter. Beat cream until softly stiff. Do not overbeat. Add ½ tsp. sugar. Fold in Amaretto and spread about one third of cream on the bottom cake layer. Place the other layer on top and coat cake smoothly with another third of the whipped cream.

Place remaining whipped cream in a pastry bag fitted with a star tube and pipe whirls of cream around edge of cake. Sprinkle with toasted almonds and refrigerate. Freezes well. Serves ten to twelve.

Alternative: Serve as a roll

When the cake is cold, carefully unroll it and spread with some of the whipped cream mixture. Reroll and place cake seam side down on a serving platter. Refrigerate until ready to serve. Decorate with remaining whipped cream and garnish with slices of fresh fruit if desired.

MUFFINS, LOAVES, COOKIES

Mini-Mental State Examination (MMSE)

Initials: ________ Date of birth: ______________ Sex: __________

Date of visit: ______________ CRF number: __________

		Points
1. Orientation in time		
Ask the patient: What is the year, the season, the date, the day, the month? Give 1 point per correctly named item (total 5 points).		..../5
2. Orientation in place		
Where are we? What is the name of the state, county, town, hospital, floor? Give 1 point per correctly named item (total: 5 points).		..../5
3. Registration		
Ask the patient whether you can test his/her memory. Tell him/her to listen carefully to the three words you will read slowly (apple, penny, table). Ask him/her to repeat the three words after you have read them once. This first recall determines the score for "registration". Give 1 point per correctly named item (total 3 points). Keep saying the words (up to 6 times) till the patient can repeat all 3.		..../3
4. Attention and concentration		
Ask the patient to count backwards starting from 100 by 7s. Stop after five subtractions. Each number must be independently compared to the prior number to ensure that a single mistake is not unduly penalised. Give 1 point per correctly made subtraction (total 5 points). Wait till after the "spelling backward" item has been completed before you give the patients final score for "attention and concentration".	..../5	
Ask the patient to spell WORLD forward. Correct if necessary before you ask him/her to spell WORLD backward. The score is the number of letters in correct order, a letter in the correct position being scored positively (total 5 points): e.g. dlrow: 5 points; dlorw: 3 points. The highest score of "counting backward" and "spelling backward" is the score assigned to the patient for "attention and concentration" (total of 5 points)	..../5	..../5

5. Recall	
Ask the patient to recall the three words you have read aloud earlier (see: 3. Registration) (total of 3 points).	..../3
6. Naming	
Show the patient a watch and a pencil. Ask him/her to name the objects. Every correct answer is given 1 point (total of 2 points)	..../2
7. Repetition	
Have the patient repeat the following: "No ifs, and, or buts". A correct repetition is given 1 point (total of 1 point). Allow only one trial.	..../1
8. 3-stage command	
Give the patient a piece of paper. Ask him/her: "Take this paper in your right hand; fold it in half and put it on the floor." Each part correctly executed is given 1 point (total of 3 points).	..../3
9. Reading	
Have the patient read and obey the following: "CLOSE YOUR EYES". Write in large letters. Score 1 point if patient actually closes his/her eyes (total of 1 point).	..../1
10. Writing	
Ask the patient to write down a sentence of his/her own choice. If the sentence contains a subject and a verb and is sensible, 1 point is given (total of 1 point)	..../1
11. Copying	
Ask the patient to copy the pentagons that are shown here. If all ten angles and intersections are present 1 point is given (total of 1 point). Tremor and rotation are ignored.	..../1

Very important instruction: All documents concerning the patient's present testing (e.g. written sentence, copied pentagons, ... should be kept in your patient file, properly dated and identified, so that they can be checked as source documents by the sponsor of the trial and by regulatory authorities.

APRICOT LOAF

Great for any occasion.

1 cup finely chopped dried apricots
1 cup warm water
2 cups unsifted flour
1 cup sugar
2 tsps. baking powder
1 tsp. salt
¼ tsp. baking soda
2 tbsps. butter or margarine
1 egg, beaten
½ cup orange juice
½ cup chopped walnuts
½ cup icing sugar
2 tbsps. milk

Preheat oven to 350° F. Soak apricots in warm water for about 15 minutes. Drain, reserving ¼ cup liquid. In a large bowl, combine flour, sugar, baking powder, salt and baking soda. Cut in butter till mixture resembles coarse crumbs. Combine egg, reserved apricot liquid, and orange juice. Add this mixture plus drained apricots and walnuts to flour mixture. Stir enough to moisten dry ingredients. Spread in greased 9" x 5" loaf pan. Bake in 350° F oven for 55 minutes or till toothpick inserted in center comes out clean. Cool in pan 10 minutes. Remove from pan and cool on rack. Combine icing sugar with milk until smooth. Spread on top of loaf.

BRAN OR WHEAT GERM MUFFINS

Mother got this recipe from her friend Georgina Watson.

¾ cup flour
3 tsp. baking powder
½ tsp. baking soda
1 cup brown sugar
1¾ cup wheat germ or bran
¾ cup milk
2 eggs
¼ cup oil

Mix dry ingredients. Beat eggs and add to dry ingredients, mixing in milk and oil. Grease 12 muffin tins and pour in batter. Bake at 400° F oven for 15 minutes.

Optional: You can add ½ cup raisins or blueberries if desired.

Early in 1997 Father began correspondence with the Geriatric Psychiatry Outreach Team at a local Elder Health Care Centre, in order that their department could commence a file on Mother. Early in 1997 Mother's scores on the mini-cognitive test dropped sharply. On January 26, 1997 her score was 25 out of 30. On March 25, 1997 her score was 20 out of 30. On April 21, 1997, her score was 18 out of 30.

JACONY COOKIES

These tasty treats can be frozen.

2 cups brown sugar
½ cup butter
½ cup margarine
2 eggs, well beaten
¼ tsp. salt
1 tsp. vanilla
2 cups oatmeal or rolled oats
1 cup coconut
2 cups flour
1 tsp. baking powder
1 tsp. baking soda

Cream butter, margarine, and sugar. Add beaten eggs, salt and vanilla. Sift flour and mix with remaining ingredients. Mix all together and roll into little balls. Flatten with wet fork on lightly greased cookie sheet. Bake at 350° F till brown.

ORANGE DATE BREAD

Great right out of the oven. Slice and spread with butter.

1 cup sugar
2 tbsps. butter
1 egg
½ cup orange juice
1 tbsp. grated orange rind
½ cup hot water
½ cup chopped walnuts
1 cup finely chopped dates or currants
1 tsp. baking soda
2 cups sifted flour
1 tsp. baking powder
1 tsp. salt

Preheat oven to 350° F. Cream sugar and butter. Stir in egg and beat well. Combine dates, orange juice, rind, hot water and baking soda in a bowl. When cool add to first mixture. Sift flour, baking powder and salt and blend in. Stir in nuts. Pour into greased 9" x 5" loaf pan and bake at 350° F for one hour.

ORANGE MUFFINS

I make these the night before and serve for breakfast.

1 whole orange, chopped
½ cup raisins
½ cup melted margarine
1 tsp. baking soda
¾ cup white sugar
½ cup orange juice
1 egg
1½ cups flour
1 tsp. baking powder

Preheat oven to 400° F. Mix orange, orange juice, and raisins in food processor. Add egg and melted margarine into the processor. In a separate bowl, mix together flour, baking soda, baking powder, and sugar. Pour the contents of the food processor into the bowl and stir well. Place in 12 muffin pan. Bake at 400° F for 15 minutes.

PINEAPPLE ZUCCHINI BREAD

Sweet pineapple and fresh zucchini blend into an amazing loaf.

3 eggs
1¾ cups sugar
1 cup salad oil
1¾ cups grated raw zucchini
1 can (10 oz) crushed pineapple, drained
3 cups flour
1 tsp. salt
1 tsp. baking soda
¼ tsp. baking powder
1½ tsps. cinnamon
¾ tsps. nutmeg
1 cup chopped nuts

Preheat oven to 350° F. Beat eggs till light and fluffy. Add sugar and continue beating until blended. Stir in salad oil, vanilla, zucchini, and pineapple. Sift dry ingredients, and stir into egg mixture along with nuts. Turn into two greased 9" x 5" x 3" loaf pans. Bake at 350° F for 50 minutes or until tests done. Remove from pan. Cool on rack. Chill before slicing.

RAISIN BRAN PEANUT BUTTER COOKIES

This came from our former next door neighbor, Doris Mattick.

1 cup sifted flour
½ tsp. baking powder
¾ tsp. baking soda
¼ tsp. salt
½ cup soft butter
½ cup peanut butter
½ cup brown sugar, firmly packed
½ cup sugar
1 egg
1 cup raisin bran flakes

Preheat oven to 375° F. Sift together flour, baking powder, baking soda, and salt. Blend butter, peanut butter, and white and brown sugar. Add egg and beat well. Add sifted dry ingredients and raisin bran flakes. Mix well. Shape into 1 inch balls. Place 2 inches apart on ungreased baking sheets. Flatten with tines of fork. Bake at 375° F about 10 minutes or until set but not hard. Allow to harden on baking sheet a few minutes before removing. Makes about 4 dozen cookies.

SCONES

Serve warm from the oven with butter.

3½ cups flour
1 tbsp. baking powder
7 tbsps. sugar
1 tsp. salt
¾ cup butter
¾ cup milk
3 eggs

Preheat oven to 425° F. Sift dry ingredients. Cut chilled butter into mixture. Beat eggs, adding to milk. Combine flour mixture and milk mixture. Flour a cutting board and roll scone to ½ inch thickness. Using cutter, or bottom of small glass, cut out scones. Should make about 15 scones. Place on greased cookie sheet and bake in 425° F oven for 15 to 20 minutes.

SCOTCH DROPPED SCONES

The Scotch version resembles mini pancakes.

¾ cup flour
1 level tsp. cream of tartar
½ tsp. baking soda
½ cup milk
2 tbsps. sugar
1 egg
pinch of salt

Sift flour, cream of tartar, baking soda, and salt. Stir in sugar and make a well in the center dropping in egg with a little milk. Mix well, adding rest of milk to make a smooth batter. Use tablespoon to pour batter onto greased griddle and cook at medium heat about one minute each side. Yields about 20 little pancakes.

SHORTEST SHORTBREAD

Melts in your mouth! Freezes well.

1 pound butter
3½ cups all purpose flour
1 cup fruit sugar
½ cup rice flour

Preheat oven to 325° F. Beat butter, then add sugar. Mix flours and add to mixture. Pat dough on cookie sheet and press down to form squares. Bake at 325° F for 30 to 40 minutes until lightly golden.

In May, 1997 Mother became part of a test study at St. Vincent's Hospital in Vancouver for a new drug called Galantamine. This was an out-patient program, a double blind study where neither the patients nor the doctors knew who was taking the real drug or who was taking the placebo. After six months, all patients would receive the real Galantamine, regardless of what they had been previously receiving. The following is part of St. Vincent's release form:

Galantamine is a new medication whose action suggests it would be helpful in improving memory and other intellectual functions in patients suffering from a dementing illness such as Alzheimer's. Galantamine increases the amount of acetylcholine (a chemical important in the function of some nerve and brain cells) in the brain by partially blocking an enzyme that breaks down the acetylcholine (ie. it's an anti-cholinesterase). In Alzheimer's Disease brain cells that use acetylcholine die and are lost. By using anti-cholinesterase medicines such as Galantamine it is hoped that the activity of the remaining acetylcholine-using brain cells can be boosted, relieving some of the Alzheimer's Disease symptoms.

JAMS

FREEZER STRAWBERRY CURAÇAO JAM

Spread over hot buttered toast, or use as a topping for ice cream.

4 cups strawberries
2 tbsps. Curaçao or other orange liqueur
4 cups sugar
¾ cup water
1 box regular Certo powdered fruit pectin

First prepare strawberries. Stem and thoroughly crush. Measure two cups into a large bowl. Add liqueur.

To Make Jam: Thoroughly mix sugar into fruit. Let stand 10 minutes. Combine water and powdered Certo in a small saucepan. Bring to a boil and boil one minute, stirring constantly. Stir into fruit. Continue stirring about 3 minutes. A few crystals will remain. Ladle quickly into jam jars or freezer containers. Cover immediately with tight fitting lids. Let stand at room temperature until set (may take up to 24 hours).

Store in the refrigerator for up to 3 weeks. Otherwise freeze as soon as its set.

Makes about 5 cups.

MONK'S MARMALADE

Toast tastes better when topped with this tangy marmalade.

1 large grapefruit
1 lemon
2 large oranges
5 lbs. sugar
4 pints water

Wash fruit. Cut into small pieces and chop in blender, or food processor, pips and all. Put in pan with water. Bring to a boil and add sugar and boil until set, about half an hour to 45 minutes. Keep stirring from time to time. Makes 10 pounds.

ACTIVITIES

It is challenging to keep the person with Alzheimer's Disease occupied and entertained during the day. Normal routines can help fill the day, such as making the bed, putting away laundry, and helping in the kitchen, but you have to keep in mind the abilities the patient has. The patient enjoys active participation and feeling useful. Choose activities that the patient still retains the skills and abilities to accomplish. Watering plants, grooming pets, and helping bake cookies are good choices. Watch out for over watering of plants. The Alzheimer's patient may enjoy this activity so much, and not remember that they have just finished watering the plants, and water them all again. Mother killed off some cactus plants due to over watering. Flower arranging and simple crafts provide immediate success, reinforcing the patient's sense of pride and self-esteem. Think about activities they enjoyed in the past, and include these in the day. Patients of Alzheimer's Disease enjoy doing the same thing over and over again, and these activities may not be boring for them.

Daily routines form a pattern, and the person with Alzheimer's Disease becomes comfortable with the routine and knows what to expect. My mother went to a hairdresser once a week. Even after she was unable to drive, my father would drive her to the appointment.

Listening to music is soothing, and all of us respond to our favorite songs. This is also an effective way of distracting the patient's attention.

Looking at photo albums and talking about the people in the pictures can bring back pleasant memories. If your photo albums do not have the names of the people written down under their photo, now is the time to record this information. Most Alzheimer's patients are able to read, and seeing the person's name next to the picture can help them remember.

Choose simple, repetitive activities such as putting flowers in a vase, tossing a ball, looking through magazines, or simple household chores like dusting, and wiping tables. Or go outside and do some light gardening.

Seasonal activities, such as Christmas decorating are also fun for the Alzheimer's patient. They enjoy decorating the Christmas tree and putting ornaments around the house. I had my mother help me put together a mock gingerbread house. The kit I bought was put together with chocolate bars and candies. My mother was able to stick the candies onto the icing and decorate the roof and windows of the little house. She was more interested in finding out when she could eat the finished candy house and deciding who else would be allowed to eat it. I bought another kit for gingerbread men and had her help me in the kitchen. She was able to put the candies onto the gingerbread men, but ate more than ended up on the cookies.

Watching familiar video movies is a good choice. My mother watched *101 Dalmatians* over and over, never tiring of the movie. Often my Dalmatian, Katy, would sit with her on the couch and they'd watch the movie together. She loved the dogs and the scenery around London. This movie was a great distraction tool for us. Whenever Mother was agitated, we'd pop it into the VCR and she'd sit there happily watching the movie.

Mother also enjoyed simple activities such as accompanying me to walk my dog or going for a drive. It didn't matter where we drove to, a department store, grocery store, gas station, drugstore, or the mall, she enjoyed the outing. I also found taking her to a donut shop was a good way to keep her occupied for up to an hour. I'd buy her a specialty coffee such as English toffee cappuccino and a donut, and she'd be quite happy watching the other people in the shop, and commenting on the people passing by on the street.

HOLIDAYS

Caring for someone with Alzheimer's Disease is very hard work, a twenty-four hour, seven days a week job. Getting some time away is very important. Everyone deserves a holiday to rest, relax, recharge batteries, and cope better upon return. After you've made a decision to take a holiday, you have to decide whether to go away together or separately. Some caregivers feel guilty about having a holiday, especially if they are leaving the Alzheimer's patient behind, but if you run yourself into the ground looking after the patient, your own health may suffer.

Going away together you'll both be able to enjoy a holiday away from your usual routine. You won't have to make other arrangements for the patient's care, and won't have to worry about what the patient is doing while you are away. However, a person with Alzheimer's Disease may be confused and upset in a strange environment, and find it difficult to get around a strange place with unfamiliar people. Sometimes a long journey can be difficult if the Alzheimer's patient tires easily or has behavioral problems. You may be able to bring along a travel companion, a family member or close friend, who can watch the Alzheimer's patient while you get away for a few hours of sightseeing and rest.

Leaving the Alzheimer's patient behind while you go on holiday means that you can get a proper break, be less restricted in what you can do, and spend some time on yourself. You will have to make arrangements for the care of the Alzheimer's patient while you are away. The simplest is to ask a relative or friend to move in to the house while you're away, or have them take the patient to their residence. If no one is available, you can contact your local Alzheimer's society for assistance. They can often recommend a nurse or care attendant who is available to care for the patient. Make sure you and the Alzheimer's patient meet with the person first and spend time getting to know the caregiver. Your Alzheimer's society or senior's care organization can also recommend hospitals and nursing homes available for respite care for a few days to a few weeks.

Long car trips with Mother turned her into an active backseat driver. It didn't matter if the driver and/or passenger knew how to get to the destination, or were following road signs or a map. Every few minutes she would say, "I think we should just turn around and go back" or "We should pull over and ask someone for directions".

When travelling by plane with an Alzheimer's patient make sure you do not get a seat near the wing. On the last plane trip I took with Mother from Vancouver to London, England, most of the journey was in darkness. Unfortunately we were seated over the wing, and the light fixture on the wing was visible from our window. Mother was unable to comprehend the light was attached to the plane, and used that light as a reference point to judge how much distance we were traveling. We remained the same distance away from that light and she became convinced we were not moving. She called over the airline attendants to inform the plane wasn't moving. One of them tried to reason with her and tell her the plane has to either be moving forward or descending. Another flight attendant realized something was not quite right with Mother, and agreed with her that the plane was indeed sitting stationary up in the air, and he would inform the pilot right away. Mother was happy with his answer, but remained concerned every time she looked out the window and realized we still had not moved away from the light.

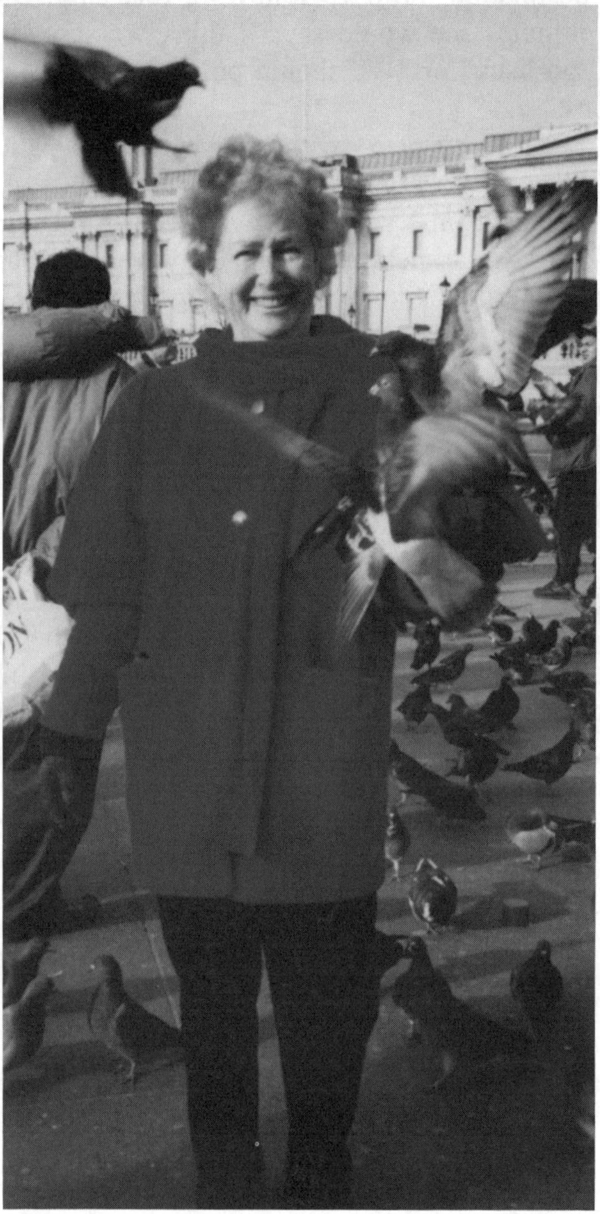

MISCELLANEOUS

TIPS FOR CAREGIVERS

To make living easier for both of you, the main thing to remember is to keep things simple. A person with Alzheimer's Disease has difficulty processing too much information at one time. Reading a menu in a restaurant became a challenge for Mother. When eating out, she would often order exactly what I was eating, right down to a diet soft drink. Other times I would make a couple of suggestions from the menu and she would make a choice.

Dressing is also a complex task for patients of Alzheimer's Disease. They have to choose the clothes, figure out which order they go on, then actually put the clothes on. For this reason many patients wear the same clothes for days, often sleeping in their clothes. The clothes are familiar to them and eliminates making a decision on what else to wear. Sometimes I would choose clothes for Mother, lay them out in the order she should put them on, and try to get the dirty clothes into the washing machine. This didn't always work. Often it was difficult to get all her dirty clothes away from her, and other times she did not like the choice of clothes I'd lain out for her. A good tip is to keep only a few clothes in the closet to make an easier decision on what to wear. The caregiver should also purchase clothes that are easy to put on.

Don't give the Alzheimer's patient too many instructions at one time as they will not remember what you have asked. While visiting my mother's sister in London, we were getting ready to go out and I asked Mother to go up to the bedroom and get her coat. A few minutes later she came back downstairs and announced that she could not find her gloves. Even though I only gave her two things to do, go to the bedroom and get the coat, she was only able to remember the first part of the instructions. She went up to the bedroom, then must have been standing around wondering why she had gone up there, finally returning downstairs empty handed. I went back to the bedroom with her, got her coat from the closet, and her missing gloves were in the pocket.

Getting Mother to take a bath became increasingly difficult. She was able to bathe unassisted, but it was hard to get her into the bath. Sometimes we would draw the water for her, put in the bath oil beads, then try to entice her into the tub. I bought a yellow rubber duck for her and kept it on the bathtub. I knew one day it would be very tough to get her into the bath, and if she was used to seeing the duck in the bathtub, then visual cues might help later on. She would make the connection that seeing the rubber duck meant it was time to take a bath. When we were able get her into the bath, the next challenge was getting her dirty clothes away from her to put into the washing machine, and have her put on fresh clothes. She was layering her clothes, so it was hard to know how many items she might have with her in the bathroom. One day my father asked me to try to get her to take a bath as it had been several days since she'd last bathed. I got the bath ready for her and tried to get her in. She did not want to take a bath, but I managed to talk her into it. I put fresh clothes in the bathroom, and asked her to pass me out all the clothes she was wearing so I could get them into the washing machine. She passed out several articles of clothing, one or two of each item, but I suspect she may have kept one or two pairs of underwear and socks in the bathroom with her. When she emerged, she was mad at me and demanded to know if I went to other people's houses and made them take baths too, and I told her yes. The thing with Alzheimer's patients is that even though they might be mad with you, they'll forget about it soon enough, and ten minutes later she was no longer mad about taking the bath.

Another thing to keep in mind, especially before going out somewhere in the car, is to remind the Alzheimer's patient to use the bathroom first. They often don't remember to go to the toilet, and regular reminders are needed to prevent accidents.

ANTIPASTO

Serve in bowl on tray surrounded by crackers.

1/3 cup olive oil
1/3 cup wine vinegar
1 bottle (1 liter) ketchup
½ bottle (285 ml) chili sauce
¼ lb. mushrooms
¼ lb. cauliflower
¼ lb. green pepper
¼ lb. red pepper
¼ lb. pickling onions
½ lb. green beans
1 jar (250 ml) pimento stuffed olives, drained & chopped
1 can (398 ml) pitted black olives, drained and chopped
¼ lb. dill cucumbers or dill pickles, chopped
1 can (198 gr.) solid white tuna, drained

Combine olive oil, vinegar, ketchup and chili sauce in a large pot. Simmer to blend flavors, about 30 minutes or longer.

Prepare all vegetables. Wash mushrooms and cut into small pieces if large. Wash cauliflower and cut into pieces, a little smaller than bite-size. Wash peppers, remove cores and cut into similar size pieces. Blanche pickling onions and skin. Chop onions if they are large. Wash beans, trim ends and cut into small pieces.

Add cauliflower, pepper and onions to vinegar mixture. Simmer 10 minutes. Add beans, mushrooms, olives and cucumbers. Bring back to boil. Add tuna, bring to boil stirring constantly. Remove from heat and cool.

Ladle into freezer cartons, leaving headspace for expansion. Cover and freeze. Makes about 10 cups.

CHEESE BALLS

Serve with apple slices dipped in lemon juice, or crackers.

1 package (250 gr.) cream cheese
3 cups grated cheddar cheese
2 tbsps. chopped green pepper
2 tbsps. chopped green onion
2 tsps. Worcestershire sauce
1 tsp. lemon juice
1 tsp. dry mustard
dash cayenne pepper
$^1/_8$ tsp. salt
1 cup chopped fresh parsley or walnuts

Beat all ingredients together except parsley or walnuts. Refrigerate for two hours. Shape into one or two balls and roll in parsley or walnuts.

How to Test Croissants For Freshness

One day Kerry and my parents stopped by a grocery store to pick up a few items. Kerry took Mother to the bakery department where he was picking out muffins. The croissants were on the shelf next to the muffins, and Mother asked him if he knew how to check croissants to see if they are fresh. She then proceeded to poke her finger through several of the croissants and as each croissant crumbled, she announced that they all passed the freshness test.

CHUCK WAGON BARBECUE SAUCE

Sauce can be used as a marinade, to baste during barbecuing, or serve as extra sauce for finished barbecued food.

1 cup ketchup
1 cup water
1 small onion, minced
1 tbsp. Worcestershire sauce
¼ cup vinegar
1 tbsp. honey
1 tbsp. brown sugar
1 tsp. paprika
1 tsps. dry mustard
1 clove garlic, minced
1 tsp. chili powder

Mix ingredients and simmer slowly together at side of grill in covered pan for 20 to 30 minutes.

For hotter sauce add dash of tobasco or cayenne pepper.

You can obtain a card similar to this from your local Alzheimer's Society. This is useful if you find yourself in an awkward public situation. You can pull the card out and let others read it.

South & Upper Fraser Valley Region

ALZHEIMER B.C.

The person with me may become confused and forgetful

Please understand any unusual behavior

HELP FOR TODAY, HOPE FOR TOMORROW

DAIQUIRI BALLS

A popular holiday treat. Freezes well.

1 cup semi-sweet chocolate chips
2½ cups crushed vanilla wafers
¼ tsp. salt
1 tbsp. grated lemon rind
2½ tbsps. lemon juice
¼ cup rum
½ cup sour cream
1 cup icing sugar, sifted
1 tbsp. cocoa, sifted
1 tbsp. grated orange rind
1½ tbsps. maple syrup
1 cup chopped pecans
icing sugar
chocolate shot

Melt chocolate chips over hot water. Allow to cool. Blend in sour cream. Combine crushed wafers, icing sugar, salt, cocoa, lemon rind, and orange rind. Blend in lemon juice, maple syrup, rum, and pecans. Mix in chocolate mixture until thoroughly combined. Refrigerate until mixture is firm enough to shape.

Shape into balls the size of walnuts. Roll in icing sugar or chocolate shot. If using chocolate shot, roll balls in this immediately after shaping as the warmth of the hands helps it stick better. Store in air tight container. Makes four to five dozen.

ESCARGOT SAUCE

What can I say about snails?

½ cup butter
1 oz. parsley
1 oz. chives
1 tsp. garlic
½ tsp. pepper
¼ tsp. nutmeg
1 can of snails
10 or 12 large mushrooms

Cook all ingredients, except snails and mushrooms, for two minutes. Add snails to the sauce and stuff into mushroom caps. Place under broiler till bubbly.

FOOD PROCESSOR ALMOND PASTE

Topping for your fruitcake, or make into small balls and roll in cinnamon.

1 cup whole blanched almonds
1 ⅓ cups sifted icing sugar
2 tbsps. water
½ tsp. almond extract

Place almonds in a single layer on baking sheet. Heat at 300° F for 10 minutes. Do not brown. Remove and cool for five minutes. Place steel blade in work bowl of food processor. Add almonds while still warm. Process about one minute, or until finely ground. Add icing sugar, water, and almond extract. Process about 15 seconds or until mixture forms a ball. Use immediately or wrap and store in freezer. Makes about one cup.

MARINARA SAUCE

Serve this zesty sauce over pasta.

2 tbsps. olive oil
1 small onion, chopped
1 can (6 oz.) tomato paste
2 tsps. basil
2 garlic cloves, minced
1 can (16 oz.) tomatoes
1 tbsp. sugar
1½ tsps. salt

About 30 minutes before serving:

In medium saucepan over medium heat combine olive oil, garlic and onion and cook until tender, about 5 minutes. Stir in tomatoes and their liquid and remaining ingredients. Reduce heat to low. Cover and cook 20 minutes or until mixture is thickened, stirring occasionally. Makes about 3 cups or enough for six side-dish serving of cooked spaghetti.

RESOURCES

CANADA

Alzheimer Society of B.C.
#20 - 601 W. Cordova Street,
Vancouver, BC, V6B 1G1
Tel: (604) 681-6530
Fax: (604) 669-6907
Web: www.alzheimerbc.org/
E-mail: info@alzheimerbc.org

Alzheimer Society of Canada
20 Eglinton Ave. W., Ste. 1200
Toronto, Ontario M4R 1K8
Tel: (416) 488-8772 1-800-616-8816 (valid only in Canada)
Fax: (416) 488-3778
Web: www.alzheimer.ca/
E-mail: info@alzheimer.ca

UNITED STATES

Alzheimer's Association
919 N Michigan Avenue
Suite 1000
Chicago, Illinois 60611
America
Tel: (312) 335-8700
Fax: (312) 335-1110
Web: www.alz.org
E-mail: info@alz.org